SHARKS STILL DON'T GET CANCER

SHARKS
STILL
DON'T GET
CANCER

DR. I. WILLIAM LANE
LINDA COMAC

Avery Publishing Group

Garden City Park, New York

The advice in this book is based on the training of, experiences of, and pool of information available to the authors. Mention of any research organization or individual researcher should in no way be construed as an endorsement of this book or of any techniques therein. Because each person and situation are unique, the editor and the publisher urge the reader to check with a qualified health professional when there is any question regarding the presence or treatment of any abnormal health condition. The publisher does not advocate the use of any particular treatment but believes the information in this book should be available to the public.

Because there is always some risk involved, the author and publisher are not responsible for any adverse effects or consequences resulting from the use of any of the preparations or procedures described in this book. Please do not use this book if you are unwilling to assume the risk. For personalized advice, please consult a physician or other qualified health professional. It is a sign of wisdom, not cowardice, to seek a second or third opinion.

Cover Design: William Gonzalez
In-House Editor: Marie Caratozzolo
Typesetter: Bonnie Freid
Figure Layouts: Nuno Faisca
Printer: Paragon Press, Honesdale, PA

Library of Congress Cataloging-in-Publication Data

Lane, I. William.
    Sharks still don't get cancer / by I. William Lane with Linda
Comac.
      p. cm.
    Follow up to: Sharks don't get cancer / I. William Lane, Linda
Comac. c1992.
    Includes bibliographical references and index.
    ISBN 0-89529-722-1
    1. Shark cartilage—Therapeutic use. 2. Neovascularization
inhibitors—Therapeutic use. 3. Cancer—Chemotherapy.
Arthritis—Chemotherapy. I. Comac, Linda. II. Lane,
I. William. Sharks don't get cancer. III. Title.
    [DNLM: 1. Neoplasms—therapy—popular works. 2. Cartilage-
-popular works. 3. Sharks—popular works. QZ 201 L265s 1996]
    RC271.S55L364 1996
    616.99'406—dc20
DNLM/DLC   96-4749
for Library of Congress   CIP

Printed in the United States of America

10 9 8 7 6 5 4 3 2 1

Contents

Acknowledgments,   xi
Foreword,   xiii
Preface,   xvii

Introduction,   1
1. A History of Shark Cartilage,   5
2. Is Anybody Really Listening?   19
3. The Media and Me,   37
4. The Government and Me,   45
5. The Scientific Community Reacts,   61
6. The Medical Establishment and Shark
    Cartilage,   79
7. Cancer Studies,   91
8. Arthritis Studies,   125
9. Administration of Shark Cartilage,   141
10. Talking to Your Doctor,   167
11. In the Marketplace,   183
    Conclusion,   199

Glossary,   209
Bibliography,   217
About the Authors,   233
Index,   235

To my friends David, Jonathan, Eva, Luis, Gilberto, Rudy,
Rand, Nabil, G.B., Tom, Ira, Jan, Patrick, Joanne, José, Roberto,
José FB, Anthony, Andre K., Mike, the countless others who stood
by me when I needed them most, and to the hundreds of patients
who have come up to me to thank me and wish me well.
Without these supporters, I could not have survived
the misinformation, negative attitudes, self-serving resistance,
and outrageous criticism directed at me from all quarters.

I.W.L.

To Pop, whose gifts live on, and Gram'Bea,
whose devotion strengthens us all.
And to my sons, Alan and Erik, with love,
and my husband, Roger, who made it all possible.

L.C.

Permissions

The quote by Philip Crews on page 5 is reprinted with permission from "Chemical Prospectors Scour the Seas for Promising Drugs" by Faye Flam. *Science* 266:1324-1325. Copyright 1994, American Association for the Advancement of Science.

The excerpts on pages 5 and 122 are reprinted with permission from "A New Phase In the War on Cancer" by Elliot Marshall. *Science* 267:1412–1415. Copyright 1995, American Association for the Advancement of Science.

The quote on page 19 is from *Gravity's Rainbow* by Thomas Pynchon, © 1973. Reprinted by permission of Melanie Jackson Agency.

The article by Tim Beardsley on pages 23–25, "Sharks Do Get Cancer," is from *Scientific American*. Reprinted with permission. Copyright © 1993 by Scientific American, Inc. All rights reserved.

The quote on page 29 is from "The Frog Treatment" by Robert Langreth. Reprinted by permission of *Popular Science* magazine, © 1993, Times Mirror Magazines Inc.

The quote on page 33 is from "Conference: Angiogenesis," *The Lancet*, June 5, 1993, pp.1467–1468. Reprinted by permission of The Lancet Ltd.

The quote from Dr. Judah Folkman on page 42 is from "Scientists Report Finding a Way to Shrink Tumors" by Lawrence K. Altman. *The New York Times*, December 29, 1994, p.1. Copyright © 1994 by The New York Times Company. Reprinted by permission.

The quote on page 141 is reprinted with permission from "Chemical Prospectors Scour the Seas for Promising Drugs" by Faye Flam. *Science* 266:1324–1325. Copyright 1994, American Association for the Advancement of Sciences.

Figure 9.1 on page 161 is from "Distribution of the Bowman Birk Protease Inhibitor," *Cancer Letters* 62:191–197, © 1992. It has been reprinted with kind permission from Elsevier Science Ireland Ltd, Bay 15K, Shannon Industrial Estate, Co. Clare, Ireland.

The quote from David Alpers on page 162 is from "Digestion and Absorption of Carbohydrates and Proteins," *Physiology of the Gastrointestinal Tract* Vol. 2, 2nd Edition, Leonard R. Johnson, ed. © 1987. Reprinted by permission of Raven Press.

Special acknowledgments to Mickey and Wally Bothum, Sister Michelle Teff, Bruce Allen, and Yoriko "Ruth" Bynum for sharing their personal accounts in this book.

Acknowledgments

A heartfelt thank you must go to Norma Sachs who answers phones, tracks information, and gives unwavering assistance with diligence, warmth, and intelligence.

Additional thanks go to all the people at Avery Publishing Group without whom this book could not reach the public. And a very special thank you goes to our editor, Marie Caratozzolo, whose eye for detail and perseverance have helped us "put our best foot forward."

Foreword

Medical history was changed forever in 1928. That year, Alexander Fleming accidentally discovered that the mold *Penicillium notatum* killed the bacterial cultures with which he was working. His surprise discovery and the introduction of penicillin forever changed the practice of medicine.

No longer an art that required the doctor to balance a patient's physical, chemical, mental, and spiritual states, medicine became a science—a science based on biochemistry. Life had been reduced to a continuous series of chemical reactions, and the idea was born that all disease could best be treated with chemicals. This philosophy has remained practically unchanged to this very day. But along with this philosophy, a disturbing trend emerged—the treatment of natural medicines and remedies with a high degree of skepticism. More emphasis is placed on the origin of medicine than on its effectiveness. As such, many very safe and effective natural products have been erroneously labeled as unscientific or unproven. No one better understands the dilemma this creates than Dr. I. William Lane.

I first learned about Dr. Lane's work with shark cartilage during a chance phone call to Dr. Robert Langer's office at the Massachusetts Institute of Technology (MIT). As editor of *Alternatives*, the monthly newsletter that focuses on breakthroughs in natural healing, I was investigating the use of shark cartilage as an effective cancer treatment. I was given the name of Dr. Lane. After a short phone conversation with the doctor, we arranged to meet at an upcoming convention on alternative cancer therapies where he was to be a guest speaker. During a private meeting following the conference, I was able to review the results of an ongoing clinical trial in Mexico in which Dr. Lane was involved.

At first I was skeptical, to say the least, about the idea of shark cartilage therapy. But the data I reviewed was nothing short of amazing. To be quite honest, I felt that Dr. Lane had either uncovered what could be one of the biggest breakthroughs in cancer treatment or a sophisticated hoax was being perpetrated.

In my work, I travel the world investigating natural treatments for practically every disease known to humankind. During my travels, I have seen my share of hoaxes. I have also seen unusually successful treatments that, for one reason or another, never seem to reach the people who need them most. Shark cartilage therapy appeared to fall into this last category. But, quite honestly, this particular situation raised more questions than it answered. For the sake of my readers and my own curiosity, it was a story I could not ignore.

How could a therapy with such promise go unnoticed for so long? Why was an individual from ouside mainstream medicine involved? Why weren't agencies like our National Institutes of Health (NIH) supporting additional research? Why was the research on shark cartilage being performed ouside the country? Why was this man spending his own money on research when billions of dollars are spent researching far-less promising therapies? As I dug deeper into the story, some of the questions were answered, others weren't.

The fact that Dr. Lane chose to take his message directly to cancer victims had not set well with many in the orthodox medical community. This, coupled with the fact that shark cartilage is a natural, nonpharmaceutical product, made the situation even more controversial.

Dr. Lane's unorthodox approaches may explain the initial skepticism surrounding shark cartilage therapy; however, it does not explain why government agencies and anticancer organizations continue to ignore his work. Hundreds, if not thousands, of surviving cancer patients are living proof that something in shark cartilage is working.

Statements claiming that not enough research has been done on shark cartilage therapy continue to surface. Unfortunately, these statements are often made by the organizations that control the research money in this country. More research must be conducted on shark cartilage. And no one would agree with this statement more than Dr. Lane. To my knowledge, Dr. Lane has encouraged and assisted in every legitimate study involving shark cartilage. But research or no research, as the saying goes, "the proof is in the pudding." If the therapy works, it will endure the test of time.

Time will be the ultimate judge of shark cartilage therapy. Dr. Lane is aware of this. On one hand, he openly welcomes legitimate scrutiny and supports continuing research. On the other hand, funds are limited and he knows all too well that those who need the therapy often have so little time. One man can do only so much. The public must demand that shark cartilage be put to the test.

Thanks to the early work of Drs. Judah Folkman, John Prudden, Robert Langer, and Anne Lee, we have several biological theories of how cartilage therapy works. Thanks to Dr. I William Lane, we now have a commercially available product and actual evidence that it is effective in treating certain cancers and other degenerative diseases. And thanks to the Food and Drug Administration, we now have approval for clinical studies in the United States. The time has come for organizations like the National Institutes of Health and the American Cancer Society (ACS) to step up to the plate and fund the necessary research.

Organizations like the NIH and ACS are nothing more than caretakers of your money, money you have provided to find a cure for cancer. No strings have been attached to this money. It doesn't matter if the cure for cancer comes from shark cartilage or some man-made prescription drug. The ultimate goal is to uncover modalities that eliminate the suffering and save lives. Shark cartilage therapy certainly appears to be one such modality. It is not a "cure-all"; no one claims that it is. It is, however, a true breakthrough whose ultimate potential remains unknown. Therein lies the importance of continuing research.

Several brilliant individuals deserve credit for the discovery, development, and commercialization of shark cartilage. But as you will see in *Sharks Still Don't Get Cancer*, the shark cartilage story is far from over. With continued support from the public and the work of brave souls like Dr. Lane, shark cartilage could prove to be one of the most important discoveries in the fight against cancer. More importantly, it is a discovery that may one day help save your life or the life of someone you love.

Meanwhile, Bill Lane continues to single-handedly spread his story of shark cartilage therapy, just as he has for over a decade. For the sake of us all, may God be with him.

Dr. David Williams
Editor, *Alternatives*

Preface

In September of 1992, *Sharks Don't Get Cancer* was published. Since then, my life has not been the same. I have been caught up in a whirlwind of meetings, travels, media interviews, and—especially—cries for help.

When I first decided to try to help people by going public with my discoveries about shark cartilage, I was fortunate enough to meet Rudy Shur of Avery Publishing Group. Committed to bringing the message of health alternatives to the general public, Rudy listened to my story, read the studies on which my work was based, and immediately saw the potentially life-saving benefits of shark cartilage. He was just as quick to see my less-than-polished writing ability, so he put me in touch with Linda Comac, a professional writer. Linda had lost an aunt and several friends to cancer. She was excited at the prospect of a potential cancer cure, as well as appalled by the lack of movement on the part of the government and traditional investigators. After many months of intense work, the three of us, in cooperation with many dedicated people at Avery, delivered *Sharks Don't Get Cancer* to the public.

Since the publication of that book, literally thousands of people around the world have begun to use shark cartilage as a cancer therapy. Thousands more have been using it to alleviate the pain of arthritis. Each week, hundreds of people call my office with inquiries. Avery Publishing Group has been deluged with such calls, as well. Daily, too, are the calls from physicians—usually stirred up by patients—wanting additional information or asking about clinical trials. When I'm not on the phone, I'm traveling around the country, talking to doctors and interested lay groups, visiting hospitals, and presenting my case to those who are best able to judge shark cartilage's efficacy. My travels have also taken me to Europe, the Far East, South America, and Cuba, where clinical trials were started in 1992, trials that have helped establish my case.

All the while, there have been people vainly trying to knock the wind out of my sails. I have had calls from people wanting to know exactly what kind of nut I am. Several media pieces have scoffed at my work. As predicted in *Sharks Don't Get Cancer*, I've been labeled by some as a charlatan and a gold digger. Yet I have funded all of my own work, unlike the very prominent investigators who often criticize me the most and who rarely, if ever, study anything without full government or corporate grants.

Where do I find the energy—and the stomach—for it all? Daily, I receive multiple "shots of adrenaline" in the form of first-hand accounts of those who claim shark cartilage has saved their lives or the lives of loved ones. Can there be a more potent motivator? The voices of those who believe I am a lifesaver have drowned out the words of those who have sought to stop me. I have weathered the storm, sailing on to arrive at what I consider a "safe harbor"—the FDA's official sanction of clinical human trials. Through these trials, the truth will at last be known.

You may be wondering why I have written a second book on the subject of shark cartilage. Well, there are several reasons. First, I felt it was important to answer some of the most common questions asked of me since the publication of my first book. I also wanted to respond to some of the troubling attitudes and reactions I have encountered. And probably most important, I felt the need to bring the public up to date on the most recent developments in the use of shark cartilage in the battle against disease.

Sharks Still Don't Get Cancer begins with a brief look at the history of shark cartilage as a therapeutic agent. Subsequent chapters allow you to share my journey—a storm-tossed journey through government, scientific, and medical establishments. A journey during which I have been buffeted by critics, bolstered by admirers, and harried by the demands of both.

Also provided are the latest research and the newest theories regarding shark cartilage's use in arthritis and cancer treatment. Perhaps most important (and exciting), actual graphic evidence of the changes affected in tumor tissue by the administration of shark cartilage is presented, evidence obtained with the help of Dr. José Fernandez-Britto. No longer am I relegated to anecdotal evidence; I now have slides from both autopsy and biopsy tissue to document the physiological effects of shark cartilage.

Later chapters focus on such areas as the administration of shark cartilage, including different techniques and dosage requirements for various conditions; how to find a physician who will work with shark cartilage; and important information regarding the proliferation of copycat products.

Throughout the book, you will find inserts illustrating the human side of my story as you meet some of those who believe they have been helped—indeed saved—by shark cartilage. You will also meet some of the scientists and physicians who have been involved in this important research and find out why they have chosen this "alternative" route.

Sharks Still Don't Get Cancer may change the way you think about shark cartilage. It may affect the way you think about health-care products or scientific research. But one way or the other, it will make you think—no bones about it.

Introduction

We've all heard the expression "living in the eye of a storm," but most of us have never actually experienced the whirlwind. I, for one, certainly never expected to. Little did I know the furor I would create.

My decision to share my findings that, based upon experimental and theoretical evidence, shark cartilage may be an effective nontoxic treatment for cancer and other degenerative diseases has certainly stirred things up. Since sharing this information with the public, I have experienced adulation and scorn, derision and respect. I have also been deluged with phone calls and letters, as well as interviews and meetings.

It could have been otherwise. I could have quietly plodded along—nagging, brown-nosing, pushing, and prodding—trying to convince physicians to try shark cartilage on their patients, trying to move government bureaucrats to approve testing. But history shows that trying to change the system from the inside rarely works. Instead, I decided to go public; after all, it is the people who are dying.

Since the publication of *Sharks Don't Get Cancer*, I have been bombarded with requests for interviews and public appearances. I have appeared on numerous television and radio shows, and have spoken before scores of cancer support groups, medical organizations, and alternative health groups. When I decided to tell my story to the public, I didn't realize how public my own life would become.

Sometimes my shark story seems more like a whale story; at times I have felt like the frustrated Jonah, trapped in the belly of the whale. But there have been some bright spots. Certainly, my television appearances on CBS's *60 Minutes* and Canada's *Market Place* were positive. I was also interviewed twice by Joan Hamburg on New York City's WOR radio network. And in April 1994, New York's FOX-5 television ran a two-night feature on my work during the 10 o'clock news. The show highlighted the patients who were involved in the clinical trials in Cuba. These people were first shown as they were at the start of the study—pale, bedridden, dying. After using shark cartilage for sixteen months, 48 percent of these patients were seen again—well, active, fully living human beings. And as my story began reaching the people, they began coming to me for more information.

During my many speaking engagements around the world—from Anaheim to Australia, from Boston to Beijing, from Tallahassee to Tokyo—it was the victims of cancer who showed up. And they showed up by the hundreds, often with stories of how shark cartilage had helped them. This is why I frequently say that the therapeutic use of shark cartilage has been patient-driven. The patients, the victims of this terrible disease, began going to their doctors with requests and questions. Their drive, their conviction, has had a major impact on the use of shark cartilage. Just consider that 29 thousand people have asked to have their names put on the mailing list for my shark cartilage newsletter. And that number continues to increase each and every day.

The impact of such a large and interested body of people has also affected the marketplace. *Sharks Don't Get Cancer* has become a best-selling book in the health arena. It has also spawned a score or more of shark cartilage products and may be responsible for the surge of interest in products from the sea in general. According to an article in *Health Foods Business*, "At the Great Earth chain of stores, supplements from the sea . . . are riding the wave of popularity generated by the news of shark cartilage." This interest has certainly been fueled by the media attention that shark cartilage has garnered. But my experiences have not all been so positive.

It has become clear to me that those who have visions that separate them from the establishment must be prepared to fight an uphill battle. For me, it has been a battle I have been proud to fight, one that has left more bright spots than wounds. Of course, the brightest spot of all has to be the Food and Drug Administration's granting of investigational new drug (IND) status for two shark cartilage products. This approval of human (Phase II) clinical trials for shark cartilage is a definite indication that the tree is starting to bend.

It is of the utmost importance that the evidence be examined, the claims be tested, and the truth be known. This is all I have ever asked. Whatever the results of the clinical trials now being conducted in the United States and many other countries, what is most important is that scientists, government agencies, and private individuals must band together to fight the *real* enemy—cancer.

My experiences since the publication of *Sharks Don't Get Cancer*—both the positive and the negative—have taught me a lot. I often feel that I've learned most from the truly excellent questions I've been asked. Those questions sometimes pointed out things I had overlooked and sometimes pointed me in new directions. Now it is time to share my experiences and the most recent information with you. Journey through the "eye of the storm" with me—I guarantee an eye-opening ride.

1.

A History of Shark Cartilage

We went through a period of 20 years when people were completely uninterested in natural products as a means of drug discovery—all the energy was in synthetic chemistry and rational drug design.

—Philip Crews
Science

- American youngsters between the ages of five and fourteen are more likely to die from cancer than from any other cause.
- In 1995, nearly 600,000 Americans died of cancer.
- Each year, more than one million Americans are diagnosed with some form of cancer.
- The overall death rate from cancer has increased in the United States over the past fifty years. In March 1995, *Science* reported, "Mortality has declined dramatically for only a few cancers, although for most, incidence is increasing faster."
- In February 1992, public health authorities at a Washington, D.C., press conference expressed "grave concerns" about

"the absence of any significant improvement in the treatment and cure of the majority of all cancers."

The battle against cancer is far from won. More than 1,400 lives are lost to the disease each day. Yet in Cuba, fourteen cancer patients involved in a clinical trial, all of whom had been under sentence of death—terminal patients who had been given less than six months to live—have already survived for more than three years with shark cartilage therapy. Furthermore, their physicians claim the therapy "dramatically improved their quality of life."

These patients had no success with chemotherapy, radiation, or surgery—all of which have side effects that can be more devastating than cancer. After all else had failed, they were treated with whole shark cartilage, a nontoxic natural product that is presently categorized as a food supplement. And these patients are not alone; thousands of patients are currently using whole, natural shark cartilage in the belief that it is shrinking their tumors, and extending and improving the quality of their lives.

The use of whole shark cartilage has proven so effective as an alternative cancer therapy that it is now being studied in human clinical trials conducted under the auspices of the United States Food and Drug Administration (FDA). Needless to say, these clinical trials were not approved by the FDA overnight or without compelling evidence. Nor was shark cartilage's development merely a fortuitous accident. The use of whole shark cartilage as an effective treatment for cancer rests upon theories that have been researched in the United States since the nineteenth century. The American people—cancer victims and government authorities alike—in large part did not know about this research until my work was brought to their attention by CBS' *60 Minutes* broadcast in February 1993.

And cancer is not the only disease for which we have been fighting a losing battle. For instance, the only treatments currently available for osteoarthritis are pain killers— which offer only symptomatic relief, are fraught with dangerous side effects, and are not even totally effective—or joint replacement. Each year, approximately 600 thousand knees, hips, and shoulders are replaced.

Over the last several years, basic science and clinical research studies have revealed that cartilage—primarily shark but also bovine (cow)—may have a beneficial effect on both cancer and arthritis, as well as on other diseases. Experimental evidence indicates that shark cartilage may act as a cancer therapy by curtailing the formation of new blood vessels. Cancer cells grow rapidly and require substantial amounts of nutrients, which must be supplied by a blood network. If the blood supply to these cells is modified, tumor growth can be affected. Motivated by these observations, I sought clinical trials on the safety and efficacy of shark cartilage. Thwarted somewhat by the scientific community and by prohibitive costs in the United States, I went first to Brussels and then to Mexico and Cuba.

THE THEORY UNFOLDS

When I became involved in shark cartilage research, I learned that it had all really started in the 1970s. At that time, Judah Folkman, M.D., of Children's Hospital and Harvard Medical School, was working on a hypothesis about the nature of tumors. During his studies with animals, Dr. Folkman noted that tumors implanted in isolated organs—organs maintained *in vitro* (outside the body in artificial environments)—grew to only a few millimeters in diameter. The same tumors implanted in mice grew rapidly, eventually killing the mice. He surmised that in living organisms, tumors develop a blood network; in a liquid medium, they do not.

Researchers eventually came to realize that in isolated organs, the layer of cells lining the capillaries (the capillary endothelium) degenerated rapidly, causing the death of the capillaries. Without these tiny blood vessels to bring them nourishment, tumors could not grow.

Then in 1971, Dr. Folkman published his now-famous hypothesis in the *New England Journal of Medicine*. His main points were:

- Tumors cannot grow without a network of blood vessels to nourish them and to remove waste products.
- Inhibiting the development of blood vessels might be a potential anticancer therapy.

The process that Dr. Folkman had investigated eventually came to be known as antiangiogenesis—*anti* meaning "against," *angio* meaning "blood," and *genesis* meaning "formation of." Formation of new blood vessels is not a common occurrence in normal adults. It occurs only during ovulation and pregnancy, in the healing of wounds and fractures, and in certain heart and/or circulatory conditions. The only other time angiogenesis—also called neovascularization—seems to occur is during the development of a tumor or other malady associated with the need for a new blood network. It appeared obvious to Dr. Folkman that a tumor could be killed by inhibiting the development of its blood vessel network. In other words, tumor growth could be arrested by stopping angiogenesis.

Believing that the halting of angiogenesis could halt tumor growth, researchers began to look for an angiogenesis inhibitor. They turned their attention to cartilage. This tough white flexible tissue attached to the bones of animals (gristle) has no blood vessels; therefore, scientists reasoned it might have an inherent mechanism for preventing the formation of these vessels. Indeed, observation of chick embryos eventually revealed that certain capillaries originally present in the embryo disappear by the fourth day of the embryo's development. The tissue in which these capillaries first appear becomes cartilage. This led researchers to believe that cartilage cells do contain a substance that inhibits vascularization. Blood vessels appear in cartilage only as a preliminary to bone formation during the fetal stage or as a preliminary to the calcification that occurs in arthritic conditions. At these times, cartilage's ability to inhibit angiogenesis seems to lose its efficacy.

An early test of the antiangiogenic capability of cartilage was conducted in the mid-1970s at the Massachusetts Institute of Technology (MIT). Robert Langer, Sc.D., and Anne Lee, Ph.D., infused an extract of calf cartilage into rabbits and mice that had been implanted with tumors. The animals exhibited no signs of toxicity, the growth of new blood vessels toward the tumors ceased, and the tumor growth stopped.

Because mammals have only a small amount of cartilage, Drs. Langer and Lee turned for their next extract to sharks, whose skeletons are composed almost entirely of cartilage. Also, the absence of fat on the shark cartilage meant that an extract of the cartilage could be prepared with a minimum of purification, eliminating the danger that the active proteins would be denatured (rendered inactive). The extract would, therefore, contain the purest possible form of the angiogenesis inhibitor. The shark cartilage extract was put in pellets that were implanted behind the corneas of rabbits. A virulent strain of carcinoma was then implanted behind the pellets. Rabbits in a control group were also implanted with tumors, but received pellets that did not contain shark cartilage.

In three separate studies, the researchers found that the shark cartilage extract inhibited angiogenesis. All of the untreated animals in the control developed large three-dimensional tumors averaging a maximum length of 6 millimeters. Animals that had received the cartilage implants had neither three-dimensional tumors nor any vascularization around the pellets. In these treated animals, the average maximum length of the blood vessels was 1.5 millimeters, 75 percent shorter than the average maximum length in the untreated animals.

Then, in 1985, Harvard-trained surgeon John Prudden, M.D., Med. Sc.D., successfully used bovine cartilage to treat human cancer patients. In Dr. Prudden's study, thirty-one patients—all of whom were selected from the large group of patients he saw—with a variety of cancers and tumors were treated using orally administered bovine cartilage as well as cartilage injected in a suspension. Over an eleven-year-period, Dr. Prudden reported that the treatment had a major inhibitory effect on cancers in patients for whom it was believed standard radiation and chemotherapy would have been of no value. All toxicity testing as required by the Food and Drug Administration proved negative, including a two-year carcinogenesis study and a sixteen-month study to determine if physical defects would be produced in offspring. Dr. Prudden was reporting tumor regression without the debilitating effects of chemotherapy, radiation, or surgery. Although Dr. Prudden's data indicates a complete response with probable or possible cure in eleven of the thirty-one cases (35 percent), this work has not, to my knowledge, been confirmed by others. (Additional information on Dr. Prudden's work with bovine cartilage and arthritis patients is presented in Chapter 7.)

Late in Dr. Prudden's study, Dr. Brian G.M. Durie, then an associate with the Department of Internal Medicine at the University of Arizona Health Sciences Center, was conducting research into the antitumor effects of bovine cartilage. He found that when bovine or shark cartilage was applied directly to tumor cells maintained in a test tube or other artificial environment, practically all of the tumor cells were killed. Dr. Durie was able to demonstrate efficacy against ovarian, pancreatic, colon, testicular, and sarcoma biopsy specimens with continuous high-dose exposure to both bovine and shark cartilage.

Dr. Langer and his associates also conducted an experiment in which they demonstrated that an extract of shark cartilage prevented angiogenesis in living organisms. They placed fertilized chick embryos in petri dishes, and the cartilage extract was

The Shark—
It's Not Just Cartilage

For more than 300 million years, the shark has roamed the seas, surviving more successfully than almost any other species. Whether it is eating, sleeping, growing, or reproducing, the shark has excelled, remaining relatively unchanged for millennia. The secrets of its success have long fascinated scientists and laymen alike, but only recently have we begun to unravel the mysteries within the shark's body.

Cartilage may prove to be the most wondrous component of the shark. It appears that a shark's cartilage plays an important role in helping to prevent the occurrence of cancer in sharks and may play a similar role for humans. The action is not a mystery; it depends on the inhibition of blood vessel growth, which is known as angiogenesis.

Although shark cartilage as an antiangiogenic may be a new concept in the marketplace, health-care products derived from sharks have been around a long time. Natural food stores have been selling shark cartilage for more than ten years, largely because of the mucopolysaccharide component, which has long been recognized as an anti-inflammatory agent. Up until World War II, shark liver oil was a major source of vitamin A, which is now synthetically produced. Now it is believed that shark liver oil can be an effective aid in cancer treatment.

Compounds found in the liver oil of sharks, primarily the cold-water sharks found off the coast of Norway and Sweden, have been characterized, researched, and used for more than three generations in the folk medicine of Scandinavian fishing villages. Fishermen use the shark liver oil from the Greenland shark or a related species to promote the healing of wounds and to treat what they call "glandular disease"—lymph node swelling.

In 1922 and again in 1926, it was reported that the active chemical substances in the liver oil of these cold-water sharks was a so-called "ether-oxygen," a type of fatty substance that differs from triglycerides by the presence of a single atom of oxygen in a unique position on the molecule. These substances are now called alkylglycerols.

Synthesized in 1930, alkylglycerols were used to treat people in the early 1950s. Astrid Brohult, a Swedish physician and researcher, demonstrated that leukopenia (decreased leukocytes and white blood cells) and thrombocytopenia (reduced platelet count), both of which result from radiation therapy, can be improved or eliminated through the administration of alkylglycerols before and during radiation treatment. She also demonstrated that patients who had received alkylglycerols before primary radiation treatment as well as throughout the course of the therapy had a significantly better survival rate than patients who had not taken the substance. The research was conducted with patients who had cervical cancer; but it is believed that similar enhancement of survival rates can be noted with other solid tumors.

It has been found that alkylglycerols play a role in stimulating white blood cell production. In fact, they are considered as essential to the production of white blood cells as iron is to red blood cell production. Alkylglycerols have been shown to elevate the production of all types of white blood cells and are, therefore, thought to be a general immune system stimulant. Alkylglycerols occur naturally in small amounts in mother's milk, in bone marrow, in the liver, and in the spleen, all of which are involved in the production of white blood cells.

Although alkylglycerols have been made available to the public, knowledge of their use is not widespread in the United States. In Germany, Dr. Hans Neiper has been reporting on the positive effects of these substances for a number of years. Patients using alkylglycerols to lessen the adverse effects of radiation therapy take six 250-mg capsules daily of processed cold-water shark liver oil. The dosage thought to stimulate the autoimmune system is two 250-mg capsules daily for adults or one daily for children.

And sharks can help us do even more than fight cancer and immune system problems. Sharks can also help us in the battle against certain harmful microorganisms. In 1993, molecular biologist Michael Zasloff, Ph.D., head of research at Magainin Pharmaceuticals in Pennsylvania, announced his discovery of an antibiotic in the stomach of the small shark known as the spiny dogfish, Squalus acanthias. He calls the antibiotic "squalamine." Dr. Zasloff says he was intrigued by the shark's hardiness. He had noted that sharks did not develop infections even after surgery. Sharks, in fact, rarely get sick although their immune system is relatively primitive.

Dr. Zasloff has demonstrated that squalamine, which is actually found in all the cells of sharks, is as potent a killer of bacteria as ampicillin but also kills other microorganisms (protozoa and fungi) by poking holes in their cell membranes. A steroid in the antibiotic is linked to a positively charged molecule; the molecule can, therefore, interact with the negatively charged membranes. Squalamine does not destroy the cells in the shark's body nor in human bodies because vertebrate cells are not negatively charged. Because bacteria cannot change their membranes, it is highly unlikely that they will become immune to squalamine, which has already been synthesized and is being tested.

The shark is beginning to look like a veritable medicine cabinet! As we learn more about the shark's success as a species, perhaps humanity will become a healthier and longer-lived species. Perhaps, too, humanity will gain increasing respect for nature's creatures.

applied to the surfaces of the embryos. Microscopic analysis repeatedly revealed that there were areas in the embryos where vascularization was being inhibited.

Subsequently, it was discovered that angiogenesis is a key factor in the development of metastatic cancers (cancers whose cells travel to and cause cancer in other sites in the body). Therefore, inhibition of vascularization (antiangiogenesis) is a means of stopping metastasis. This concept was proven by a team of Boston physicians that included Dr. Folkman and was published in a 1991 report in the *New England Journal of Medicine*. By examining surgically removed tumor tissue, the team of physicians was able to prove that when more capillaries are present in tumor tissue, the number of metastases increases. It was shown that for each 10-vessel increase in the microvessel count, there was a 1.17-fold increase in the risk of distant metastasis.

Metastasis is dependent on angiogenesis at least in part because it is easier for tumor cells to penetrate newly developing capillaries than mature vessels. Angiogenesis, therefore, provides a perfect route for tumor cells to move into the circulation, causing metastasis. In addition, the tumor cells at the metastatic site must induce angiogenesis if they are to survive; this is more likely to occur when the primary tumor is highly angiogenic.

As the research proceeded, it became apparent that although several substances other than shark cartilage have been identified as angiogenesis inhibitors (see pages 111–121), all displayed some level of toxicity and could not be used over an extended period of time. The most effective antiangiogenic agents among those listed are very difficult to synthesize. However, heparin-steroid combinations are useful as the standard by which angiogenesis inhibition can be measured.

For instance, heparin-hydrocortisone receives an index of 0.55 to 0.75 on a scale derived for evaluation of antiangiogenic activity. Pure shark cartilage powder—refined so that it contains at least 39 percent protein and less than 0.02 percent fat—receives a minimum index of 0.85 varying up to 1.1 on the high side. The potency of shark cartilage as an angiogenesis inhibitor increases with its increasing protein content. Unfortunately, the procedure originally used to evaluate antiangiogenic activity—the chicken chorioallantoic membrane or CAM assay—has proven unreliable. Current work by at least two groups—one a pharmaceutical assaying group and one a university research group—using a more reliable procedure called an endothelial cell procedure has shown that properly prepared shark cartilage is very active" as an angiogenesis inhibitor.

In an attempt to develop antiangiogenic agents that could be used in patients, investigators turned their attention to identifying the protein or proteins in shark cartilage responsible for antiangiogenesis. By 1990, at least two and possibly three of these proteins had been identified. Dr. Langer and his associates published a paper in *Science* in which they reported that they had identified a specific macromolecule derived from cartilage as a strong angiogenesis inhibitor. They called the substance cartilage derived inhibitor (CDI). In the same year, Japanese researchers reported a crude separation of a second and possibly a third protein in shark cartilage responsible for the inhibition of angiogenesis. More recently, Dr. K.P. Wong of Fresno State University (see pages 119–121) claims to have separated four proteins in shark cartilage that demonstrate antiangiogenic activity. As of this writing, however, researchers have not been able to isolate or synthesize the active substances.

Researchers have turned to the tasks of isolating and synthesizing a nontoxic antiangiogenic substance so they can get FDA approval for a drug that can be patented. In this way, researchers and the universities or companies they work for can protect themselves against competition, advertise a unique product, and recoup the estimated $359 million spent doing the testing required by the FDA. During the years involved in pursuing isolation and synthesis, hundreds of thousands will die; thousands more will suffer. To me, such research appears more profit-oriented than people-oriented.

With so many scientists devoted to this form of drug research, how much progress have we been able to make? When one looks at the latest "medical boons," it doesn't seem that much has actually been accomplished. Recently, the media has touted Tacrine, a drug that received FDA approval for the treatment of Alzheimer's disease. Marketed as Cognex, Tacrine is currently expected to help *less than half* of those suffering from Alzheimer's. In the area of cancer therapy, there's the much-publicized Tamoxafen, which was enthusiastically embraced by the medical establishment as a means of preventing the recurrence of breast cancer. Unfortunately, Tamoxafen use carries with it an increased risk of uterine cancer. Taxol, another in the long line of cancer drugs, received FDA approval at the end of December 1992. It reduced tumor size by at least half—but only in 20 to 30 percent of patients. And even those patients whose tumor size had been reduced lived an average of only nine months longer than untreated patients. Taxol also has side effects that include hair loss and numbness in fingers and toes.

Now, let's look at shark cartilage, which has never been shown to have a side effect other than occasional intestinal gas, and has reduced tumors in a large number of the patients who have used it; these patients have survival rates that currently exceed three years. Unfortunately, the percentage of survivors varies depending on the type of tumor and the disease stage at which the shark cartilage is first administered. What is consistent is an enhanced quality of life and a reduced level of pain in almost all cases. Yet the FDA strictly prohibits the marketing of shark cartilage as a cancer therapy until the therapeutic effects have been proven in controlled clinical trials. It is available only as a food supplement. Anyone selling it with the advice that it has medicinal benefits is liable to criminal prosecution, fine, and imprisonment. There is also the threat that shark cartilage may then be taken off the market completely and will no longer be available to those who are using it. Compared to Taxol, which is widely used, costs the medical system hundreds of millions of dollars, and achieves only a 20 to 30 percent success rate (with Stage III and IV cancer patients surviving an average of only a few months), shark cartilage has demonstrated noticeably better results. To date, 48 percent of the Stage IV patients involved in the Cuban study of shark cartilage have survived for three and a half years.

THE LURE OF THE SHARK

I didn't discover the information about shark cartilage over-night. I first became involved with shark cartilage in the mid-1970s. As a consultant to the government of Iran, I was asked to study the development of a fishery in the Persian Gulf where sharks are abundant. I became fascinated with sharks and their economic potential and decided to go into the shark business for myself. An associate who wanted to help me market my products introduced me to Dr. Prudden with the idea that he might want to buy the cartilage, which would be just a leftover of the planned shark business. When I met Dr. Prudden in 1983, I really didn't believe that bovine cartilage or any cartilage could achieve the wonders he claimed. But I didn't see any harm in trying the stuff; I took some of his "magic pills" to see if they'd help my bad back. They did. Within three weeks, my pain had greatly diminished and my mobility had increased. Later, I suggested that an acquaintance of mine try the cartilage preparation to relieve an arthritic condition that prevented her from lifting her arms even as high as her shoulders. After three weeks on the preparation, she was able to clap her hands easily and painlessly over her head.

Just a few months later, I heard the news on CNN: "Shark cartilage cures cancer," a report on the work of Drs. Lee and Langer at the Massachusetts Institute of Technology. Since then, I've been a man obsessed. Throughout the years, I've worked completely on my own and even funded myself, albeit with a very minimal budget compared to the pharmaceutical houses.

I worked for eight years to develop a method for processing shark cartilage without destroying its active components and received a use patent as a result. And I've done everything in my power to get physicians and researchers to try shark carti-lage on cancer patients. People who are dying simply don't have the time to wait for scientists to identify, isolate, and purify the proteins responsible for shark cartilage's antiangiogenic activity. Time can be a cancer patient's worst enemy.

IN CONCLUSION

Compassion for cancer victims should be enough to motivate investigators to work with me. And even if compassion is not "controlled" enough for researchers, the belief that a scientist's job is to find the truth should do the trick. But I feel as if I've been swimming upstream. To say I've met with a lot of resistance is an understatement.

Physicians have often been reluctant to try shark cartilage on their patients. And those physicians who do call me regarding the cartilage are often victims of cancer or have family members with cancer. Many are not aware of the facts as presented in my first book, *Sharks Don't Get Cancer*, but few are unaware of the ridicule heaped upon me by many of the most active cancer researchers—people who should know better. The negative comments of these researchers have often been echoed by government agencies, which have repeatedly thwarted my attempts to have the research move forward. A wealth of misinformation, as we shall see in the next chapter, has been disseminated by these people as well as by media representatives.

2.

Is Anybody Really Listening?

If they can get you asking the wrong questions, they don't have to worry about the answers.

Thomas Pynchon
Gravity's Rainbow

We all know that people see and hear what they want to or what they expect to. Psychologists call this *selective perception*; each person's perceptions are limited by his or her expectations. Information on shark cartilage has fallen victim to this psychological phenomenon. Some people have a preconceived notion that alternative medicine—in any form—is nothing short of quackery. Such belief undoubtedly limits their willingness to accept shark cartilage as an effective therapy, and they are simply unable to see or hear the facts. In many cases, these people—media and government representatives, scientists, and physicians—end up passing along information that is not based on the truth.

After the publication of my first book, I was at first gratified. I had taken a major step in getting the word about shark cartilage to the public. In a few cases, my critics provided reasonable, accurate, and unbiased accounts of the book and the therapy. And although some of these accounts ended on notes of skepticism, that was just fine. I certainly expected and even welcomed the challenge of fair criticism of my work. What I hadn't expected, however, were the misrepresentations and the unfair treatment my work received.

EXCLUSIONARY, SELECTIVE, AND DISTORTED VIEWS

Over the last two years, I have found myself facing a barrage of distortions, fabrications, misleading criticisms, and omissions of information. Such accounts have been published in mainstream publications and scientific works and have been seconded by researchers and clinicians. As I encountered each new instance of misinformation, my frustration increased. It seemed as if roadblocks were constantly being thrown in my path in an attempt to keep the truth from getting out. But why? What were my critics afraid of? That the public would become aware of a potential cure for cancer?

I don't think the negative responses were planned. There was no conspiracy, no sinister organization behind what was occurring. But the end result was the same: distorted accounts of important information. And I can't help but feel my work received negative treatment because much of the research was performed outside the mainstream environment. All you have to do is look at the media to see how much we rely on mainstream physicians and researchers for information. For example, *The New York Times* printed a front-page article entitled "Scientists Report Finding a Way to Shrink Tumors." This article discussed the work of mainstream researchers only; it never quoted anyone involved with shark cartilage therapy. (See page 42 for detailed discussion of this article.)

In another case, the January 3, 1996, edition of that same paper ran an article in the OP-ED section under the following banner headline: "Buying Snake Oil With Tax Dollars." The article, which was written by two professors—not of medicine, but of physics and biology—questioned the validity of the Office of Alternative Medicine (part of the National Institutes of Health) in spending money to investigate "unconventional medical practices." The article included a number of unsubstantiated claims. A few days later, two letters appeared on the editorial page in response to the article. The intent of both letters, which were written by the first and the present directors of the Office of Alternative Medicine, was to set right the misconceptions found in the article. Guess what the headline read above these two letters? "U.S. Health Agency Isn't Pushing Alternative Medicine." Whether it was intentional or not, this headline served to solidify a negative concept of alternative medicine in the minds of its readers.

Consider, too, that when New York's Eyewitness News did a segment on shark cartilage (see page 87), the only health-care professional interviewed was Dr. James F. Holland, an oncologist at Mount Sinai Medical Center. His response reflected a very narrow view of the use of this treatment. Such emphasis on mainstream medicine denies the public access to alternative approaches. People are being robbed of findings and information to which they have every right, limiting their freedom of choice.

Subtle Cases of Misinformation

When the news about shark cartilage began to catch the public's attention, questions on its use started making their way to medical columnists in newspapers and magazines throughout the country. Unfortunately, in far too many instances, these medical people responded to the readers' questions in less-than-professional ways. The following account is a prime example.

In October 1993, a rheumatologist on Long Island's North Shore responded to a query in a community paper about shark cartilage's usefulness for an arthritis sufferer. The doctor claimed that there was no reason to believe that ingesting the substance would replace worn cartilage. No one ever claimed it would! The point of shark cartilage therapy in arthritis is to reduce inflammation and stop the vascularization of normally avascular cartilage, which gives rise to calcification (see Chapter 7). No one ever stated that it would *replace* cartilage. This physician, who obviously never read my book nor attended one of my talks, could have called me or my publisher for accurate information before responding to the query. Instead, he chose to answer the question without knowing the facts. Can you see the potential damage that was done here?

In another case, a magazine printed a reader's response to a story it had run on shark cartilage. The writer of the letter was indignant. He was appalled that the editor had printed information that was misleading and untrue, claiming that a recent study had shown that shark cartilage was absolutely useless. My immediate thought was, "What study?" Strange that I have never heard of such a study. Strange, too, that the research team or sponsoring organization of the study was never mentioned. I wonder why the magazine editor never asked for details of this so-called study or some verification that it even existed. How "misleading" is that? Unfortunately, when the general public reads such misinformation, it has a tendency to believe it or, at the very least, be confused by it.

People's ability to learn the truth about shark cartilage has also been compromised through simple omission. A November 1994 issue of *Science* included an article entitled "Chemical Prospectors Scour the Seas for Promising Drugs." Guess what was not mentioned? You've got it—shark cartilage. Although the article begins with a discussion on the pulverization of a lobster and the subsequent soaking of the material in an attempt to produce extracts that can be tested against a number of human tumors, no mention is made of any research with sharks. This is most surprising because of a total of six anticancer compounds discussed at length in the article, only one had reached the clinical trial phase in the United States. Two had clinical trial applications pending, two were preclinical, and one was in clinical Phase II in Canada. Certainly, shark cartilage's position on the "clinical ladder" should have merited its inclusion in this article. I cannot help but feel that the author and/or editor believed shark cartilage was too entrenched in alternative medicine to be mentioned in a journal of pure science.

The scientific community has a long history of ignoring alternative therapies. Just think about reactions to the ancient arts of acupuncture and herbal healing. Unfortunately, when such reactions appear in print, readers may end up questioning the validity of alternative medicine.

A Glaring Case of Misinformation

I think the most frustrating piece of misinformation in response to my work came from *Scientific American*, probably one of the most highly respected voices of science in the United States. Founded in 1845, *Scientific American* has a worldwide circulation of one million readers.

In response to my first book, *Scientific American* printed an article by Tim Beardsley entitled "Sharks Do Get Cancer." As I read the article (reprinted in its entirety below), I couldn't believe my eyes:

> *Sharks Do Get Cancer*
> *Cartilage cure relies on wishful thinking*
>
> *A pseudoscientific myth holds that sharks don't get cancer. Indeed, that proposition is the title of a book by I. William Lane and Linda Comac promoting shark cartilage as a "break-through in the prevention and treatment of cancer and other*

degenerative diseases." The CBS television program "60 Minutes" enthusiastically picked up the idea earlier this year.

Unfortunately, John C. Harshbarger, director of the registry of tumors in lower animals at the Smithsonian Institute in Washington, D.C., says he has records of at least 20 cases of cancer in sharks. The registry, which is supported by the National Cancer Institute, includes shark cancers that originated in the cartilage, as well as cancers of the kidneys, liver and blood cells. (Harshbarger says data do not exist to determine whether sharks get cancer more or less often than do other creatures.)

In their book, Lane and Comac cite an article about cartilage by Arnold I. Caplan, a biologist at Case Western Reserve University, published in this magazine in October 1984. Caplan had noted that cartilage seemed to contain substances that inhibit the growth of blood vessels and speculated that such substances might someday be used to prevent tumors from establishing the blood supply they need to grow.

Caplan was right: cartilage does indeed contain inhibitors of blood vessel growth, or antiangiogenesis factors. Some have been isolated and are now in clinical trials for treatment of a variety of cancers as well as stomach ulcers. But Caplan says he is "appalled" by Lane and Comac's effort to promote shark cartilage as a treatment. "This is an extreme interpretation of the data," Caplan complains. Moreover, he adds, "There's nothing special about sharks. Why not eat pigs' knuckles?"

Caplan is not the only investigator troubled by the shark cartilage craze. Judah Folkman, an angiogenesis researcher at Harvard Medical School, states firmly that there is no evidence in any controlled study that ingesting cartilage can treat cancer. What is more, he notes, on the basis of what is known, "a patient would have to eat hundreds of pounds of cartilage" to have any chance of experiencing an effect. Folkman says he has been trying for years to dissuade Lane from using his name to promote a shark cartilage product.

> *Carl A. Luer, an investigator at the Mote Marine Labora-*
> *tory in Sarasota, Fla., who appeared on "60 Minutes," is also*
> *dismayed that his work on antiangiogenesis factors is being*
> *used to promote shark cartilage. "I feel our factor is a protein*
> *and can't be absorbed," he states. Some tropical shark popu-*
> *lations, he says, are already depleted by overfishing.*
>
> *The National Cancer Institute has examined some cases*
> *of supposed improvements in patients treated with shark*
> *cartilage, but the data "did not show solid evidence of clinical*
> *activity," according to Mary S. McCabe, a clinical trial or-*
> *ganizer at the institute. Still, enthusiasts are persevering.*
> *Charles Simone, a physician in private practice in New Jersey,*
> *maintains that a few of his patients have responded favorably.*
> *But even he warns against self-medication. Much of the shark*
> *cartilage now on sale in health food stores, he says, is "bogus*
> *stuff."*
>
> *—Tim Beardsley*

My frustration with this article began with its first line: "A pseudoscientific myth holds that sharks don't get cancer." Beardsley, who supposedly had read my book, was essentially saying that I had lied, since some sharks *do* get cancer. Had he actually read the book, he would have seen my explanation for the title in the preface. I clearly stated on page xviii, "I must admit that *some* sharks do get cancer. The number is, however, insignificant; and while *ALMOST No Sharks Get Cancer* might have been a bit more accurate, it would have been a rotten title." Furthermore, on page 4 of the book, I gave specific information on the number of sharks that do, indeed, get cancer—"The total number of shark tumors is less than a fraction of 1 percent of the total tumors reported for all fish."

In addition, some of the prominent investigators whose works were cited in my first book were quoted in Beardsley's article. One in particular seems to have taken umbrage at my position. Arnold I. Caplan, Ph.D., whose comprehensive 1984 article on cartilage was referred to in my first book, says he is "appalled" and claims that *Sharks Don't Get Cancer* is "an extreme interpretation of data." It appears that Dr. Caplan, like so many of my critics, did not even read my book. In the aforementioned *Scientific American* article, he is quoted as saying, "There's nothing special about sharks. Why not eat pig's knuckles?" Although I cannot tell you why you shouldn't eat pig's knuckles, I can refer Dr. Caplan and you to the overwhelming evidence for shark cartilage's therapeutic value as cited in *Sharks Don't Get Cancer*.

For instance, in 1983, Drs. Lee and Langer of MIT published, "Cartilage Contains Inhibitors of Tumor Angiogenesis" in *Science*. I don't think the peer reviewers at *Science* or the scientists themselves will appreciate the research's being reduced to the level of "nothing special." Furthermore, Dr. Caplan may not be aware that in 1990, Japanese investigators reported in *Cancer Letters* that they had identified two proteins in shark cartilage that are active angiogenesis inhibitors. I have read nothing in scientific or lay journals about pig's knuckles.

The kind of information that appears in the *Scientific American* article may explain why William Jarvis, president of the National Center Against Health Fraud, has been quoted as saying that there is no reason to believe shark cartilage works. "Sharks get cancer. They even get tumors of the cartilage." Apparently, he didn't read my first book either. But let's get down to numbers.

In the *Scientific American* article, John C. Harshbarger, director of the registry of tumors in lower animals at the Smithsonian Institute, cites at least twenty cases of cancer in sharks. That's twenty cases since the registry's inception in 1965, less than one case a year, indicating a cancer rate for sharks of about one in one million. I stand by my contention that the number is insignificant. But that isn't even the issue. The only relevant question is, "Does shark cartilage work?" I believe it does. My reasoning is based on the sound theoretical framework that came out of Harvard and on the subsequent experimental evidence out of the Massachussetts Institute of Technology. I stand by Dr. Caplan's contention, quoted in my first book: "Perhaps a factor derived from cartilage, applied to a growing tumor, could throttle its blood supply and thus bring on its death." Why is he so upset at my attempt to prove him correct?

I knew the damage that the *Scientific American* article could do to the work in which I was involved. I immediately sent the following reply to the magazine's editor:

November 16, 1993
Jonathan B. Piel, Editor
Scientific American

*In the article entitled "Sharks Do Get Cancer. Cartilage cure relies on wishful thinking" (**Scientific American**, October 1993, page 25), Tim Beardsley presented a one-sided and negative report on shark cartilage and its medical potential that denied your readers a balanced and informed account of the shark cartilage story.*

If your magazine had opted to present a complete story on shark cartilage research, your readers would have learned that 15 of 29 terminal cancer patients that took part in a human clinical trial in Cuba, treated only with shark carti-lage, are still alive and well after approximately 15 months, when, by definition, all should have died within 6 months. Your readers would also have learned that the FDA recently granted approval to commence a Phase II clinical investiga-tion to evaluate the safety and effectiveness of dry shark cartilage—the same cartilage product used in the Cuban study—in reducing tumor size and improving quality of life in advanced prostate and breast cancer patients. This is one of the first times that the FDA has approved such a study using a natural product.

Finally, your readers would have learned that at a recent meeting of the World Congress of Anatomic and Clinical Pathology, histologic slides from both autopsy tissue and biopsy tissue from patients in the Cuban study, taken before and after shark cartilage treatment, clearly showed the anti-tumor effect of shark cartilage therapy.

***Scientific American** has always been known for thorough and honest reporting. In this case, I found Tim Beardsley's article to be so one-sided as to bring discredit to your magazine. If you are interested in doing a full review of shark cartilage therapy, I and those with whom I work would be happy to provide you with all relevant data and information.*

I anxiously await your reply.

Sincerely,

I. William Lane, Ph.D.

A few days later I received a response—a one-sentence reply that simply defended the author of the article, Tim Beardsley. It said:

November 18, 1993
Dr. I. William Lane
Cartilage Consultants, Inc.

Dear Dr. Lane:
We stand by Mr. Beardsley's story (and shy away from uncontrolled clinical trials).

Sincerely,

Jonathan Piel

I was dumbfounded! The potential for an effective treatment presented in *Sharks Don't Get Cancer* deserved some real attention, but all *Scientific American* gave it was a complete distortion of the truth. Adding to my frustration was the fact that the journal would not give me any space to respond to the inaccuracies of its article. Unfortunately, this behavior may be indicative of the attitude of many major scientific journals—not only can they get away with printing misinformation, they don't really care about the consequences. How many potential cures have fallen by the wayside when research funding dried up because of an unfair article in a major journal?

It is also interesting to note the absence of complaints when members of the establishment say, "Sharks don't get cancer." In August 1993, *Popular Science* reported on the development of squalamine, an antibiotic derived from sharks (see *The Shark—It's Not Just Cartilage*, beginning on page 11). Writer Robert Langreth noted, ". . . sharks, as far as researchers can tell, don't get cancer." He went on to quote John Forrest, Ph.D., a researcher from Yale Medical School, "Every summer for the past 22 years I've operated on [dozens] of sharks, and I have never seen one with a tumor."

DECEPTIVE CRITICISM

Over the years, critics of scientific work have developed stock responses to non-mainstream breakthroughs. Initially, these responses may sound impressive, but once analyzed, many of these comments are really quite weak. And, as you will see, these criticisms are often misleading and simply do not address the pertinent issues.

The Matter of Peer Review

According to the critics, in order for a scientific work to be taken seriously, it must first appear in an established peer-review journal. Here I am struggling to get the financing to underwrite studies, to get the government's approval to conduct trials, to get the public's attention, and people tell me I can't be taken seriously until I stop what I'm doing and get published through "peer review."

Traditionally, scientific findings are published in journals that require the articles be reviewed by other scientists. The "studies must meet a host of requirements to be considered valid." As you'll see in Chapter 3, *60 Minutes* was far more thorough than any peer-review journal. Furthermore, the peer-review system has many failings. Consider, for instance, that peer reviewers are often people who have vested interests in the scientist whose article is before them. Some of the author/scientists sit on panels that have control over funding. Some have jobs to offer. And someday, the reviewer will have an article he wants published. It's one heck of an old-boy network.

Science, perhaps the best known and most widely read of the peer-review journals, has often been called the "Scientist's house organ." If scientists are all members of the same house, do outsiders stand much chance of getting in?

The biggest failing of peer-review articles is that they do not guarantee the integrity of the author/scientist and, therefore, cannot guarantee that the information is accurate. Recent scandals surrounding falsified data in studies comparing the benefits of lumpectomies with those of mastectomies revealed that peer review is simply not a great watchdog (see *Peer Review Misses the Mark* beginning on page 64).

It's actually funny that one researcher is quoted as saying that I need to publish in scientific journals so that people can judge my findings "for themselves." The fact is, most people don't read those journals or even know what's in them. The information about angiogenesis and shark cartilage had been buried in that type of publication for twenty years. While the scientists labored in their labs and reported in peer-review journals, tens of thousands of people continued to die.

Don't misunderstand. I certainly don't mean to minimize the work of those who have been published in scientific journals. What I am saying, though, is that a person shouldn't be crucified for not being published in them.

I did go to the public, but I did it in a book, and I did it on *60 Minutes* and a host of other broadcasts. The researcher I just mentioned was right; people should judge for themselves. After all, the public's tax dollars support the research to the tune of almost $2 billion a year. I felt compelled to write my first book because I wanted people to know what had been going on in the ivory towers of academia. Until the book was published, the information had appeared only in scientific publications. Now, *Sharks Still Don't Get Cancer* tells the story of what happened once the public found out.

The Language Maze

In some instances, people—many who have vested interests—confuse the issue of shark cartilage's effectiveness by masking the truth. The misuse of language is one way in which this is done.

One tactic that tends to instantly invalidate a therapy is use of the terms "no proof" or "no evidence." Consider that some scientists say there is no evidence that the proteins in the cartilage could have an effect if taken by mouth or enema. It seems to me that fourteen people in Cuba, eight in Mexico, and those Americans discussed in this book constitute at least *some* evidence.

Here's another example of the use of language to confuse: The author of an article in *Scientific American* writes, "There is no proof that [shark cartilage] is effective." I must respond by saying that there may not be irrefutable proof, at least not yet, but there is certainly enough evidence to indicate that further research is warranted. That's all I have ever asked—that shark cartilage therapy gets an honest shot to prove itself. The truth is the jury is still out; trials and tests are still going on; no verdict has yet been handed in.

There is a world of difference between the terms "un-proven" and "disproven." At this time, the effects of shark cartilage are considered "unproven"; therefore, the product cannot legally be sold as a drug in the United States. Something "unproven" may one day, in fact, be "proven." On the other hand, when something has been "disproven," the facts are all in, the truth is known. When discussing shark cartilage, "un-proven" signifies that all of the facts are not yet in.

Shark cartilage therapy is sometimes referred to as an "uncon-ventional treatment." The Office of Technology Assessment, an agency that serves Congress, defines unconventional cancer treat-ments as "those treatments that fall outside the bounds of main-stream medicine and have not been proven safe or effective by scientific standards that balance benefit and risk." This is in con-trast to experimental therapies, which are defined as "new prod-ucts under investigation or approved products being tested for new uses." As of this moment, shark cartilage is neither disproven nor unconventional; with the granting of an IND, it became "a new product under investigation" (see page 48).

Are scientists deliberately using misleading terminology when discussing shark cartilage? Jerry Olarsch, president of Naturopathic Research Laboratories, believes that mainstream scientists seek to protect the establishment. He feels that they have a motive for discrediting shark cartilage therapy; they want to protect the profits of the pharmaceutical companies that fund their universities' research (see *Peer Review Misses the Mark* beginning on page 64).

Avoiding the Issues

There is another way in which the public is commonly misled—many critics simply don't address the issues. Instead, some resort to name-calling or arguing by absurd analogy. For in-stance, one researcher said, "I guess I just don't understand the difference in what he's [Lane] doing and in all of a sudden giving people lots of orange juice or lots of apples or sawdust." Of course, there's a difference. I've backed my claims with evidence that I have put before you.

In addition, no one denies that antiangiogenic agents can be vital weapons in the war against cancer. Quite the opposite is true. Many scientists are currently engaged in research to identify angiogenic agents that can be used therapeutically. According to the prestigious British medical journal *The Lancet*, "progressive solid tumour [sic] growth is known to be angiogenesis dependent. . . . It seems that the potential for therapeutic intervention by inhibiting or promoting angiogenesis is being realized." Very recent work on angiogenesis and cancer has appeared on the front page of *The New York Times* (see page 42), and almost monthly, articles on angiogenesis research appear in such important journals as *Science*. But no one in any of these articles is saying anything about sawdust. And no one is saying anything "all of a sudden." Research into cartilage as an antiangiogenic agent began decades ago.

Scientists are not the only people whose words demonstrate that their preconceived notions may be keeping them ignorant of my work. William Jarvis of the National Center Against Health Fraud has said of shark cartilage, "One of the sure signs of a quack remedy is that it claims to treat all kinds of cancer. Another clear sign is that it claims to cure a wide variety of conditions." I have always said that shark cartilage will not affect cancers that are not angiogenesis-dependent. There is no reason to assume that it will work on leukemia, Hodgkins, or other blood cancers. In a similar vein, I have made no claims that shark cartilage will cure a "wide variety of conditions." What has been said is that *theoretically* any disease that is the result of angiogenesis, that depends on the proliferation of capillaries, should be affected by an antiangiogenic agent such as shark cartilage.

It is interesting that the word "quack" seems to surface

when my work is being discussed. The word never appeared when the September 1992 issue of *Biotechnology* discussed "Angiogenic and Angiostatic Drugs" as a means to fight conditions as diverse as "a wide variety of cancers," inflammation-producing diseases such as arthritis and autoimmune psoriasis, and diabetic retinopathy. No one called Dr. Folkman a quack when he said that antiangiogenesis could benefit patients suffering from thirty to forty related diseases. And *The New York Times* referred to angiogenesis research as a possible "magic bullet" against cancer.

Another interesting ploy is criticizing research that does not involve double-blind studies. Such studies involve administering two substances: the one being tested and a placebo such as sugar water. Neither the doctors administering the substance nor the patients receiving it know which is which. Every doctor that I have talked to at the FDA will tell you that if you're working with terminal patients, you don't need a double-blind study. According to these FDA physicians, nearly all of the patients will die, and keeping even 10 percent of them alive would be extraordinary. I would also like to point out another interesting fact. According to a 1978 government assessment of the efficacy and safety of medical technologies, published by the Office of Technology Assessment, 80 to 90 percent of mainstream medical procedures in the United States have never been subjected to controlled studies of any kind. The procedures were accepted simply because they worked. But the issue of double-blind studies continues to haunt me.

My critics want me to be cautious like other researchers. They say my studies are based on anecdotal evidence, and I stand to make a profit. Yet many of these critics are the scientists who for years refused to participate in studies that would generate the necessary scientific evidence. And berating me for making a profit at best avoids the real issue of whether or not shark cartilage works.

The fact is, my mission is to get others to do the studies—

including double-blind—and have their results published. If I have the opportunity to be involved, I will. But I will tell you this: Whether or not an article appears in a peer-review journal will not make the findings about shark cartilage any less important. Those findings will stand on their own; whether a handful of people choose to ignore it is not my business. The public has the right to know what is going on. And it is up to the people to make the necessary choices.

Again, I am not afraid of criticism. I believe very strongly in my work, and I have no trouble defending it. The problem lies in the unfair accusations with which I have to deal. Whether planned or not, the types of criticism discussed here cause me to spend precious time defending myself and my work against non-relevant issues. I am forced to waste time, rather than use it to focus on the heart of the matter.

IN CONCLUSION

I know we live in a "relatively" free society, and that the examples of misinformation described in this chapter come with the territory. The point I'd like to make, however, is that the responsibility of making the right choices falls squarely on your shoulders. I know that I am prepared to continue the fight for the use of shark cartilage as a potential treatment against cancer and certain other diseases and conditions. You must, therefore, be prepared to listen closely to what is really being said or not said. Do not be afraid to question the "so-called" experts in their judgments. For the sake of us all, allow this treatment to be proven right or wrong on the facts, not on the misplaced criticisms of others.

3.

The Media and Me

A lot of people simply can't believe that the deliberate suppression of lifesaving, valid therapies—especially cancer therapies—is possible in modern America. Unfortunately, they are dead wrong.

—Richard Walters
Options

T he word "shark" seems to be a magnet that draws the public's attention, conveying images of mystery and terror upon which the media is only too willing to trade. Shark cartilage, too, has drawn an abundance of media attention. But it hasn't always been that way. And the coverage hasn't always been positive.

When I first discovered that shark cartilage might halt the growth of tumors, I set out to get people interested in conducting the necessary research. Not only did I approach scientific investigators, I also looked for backers, people who could put up the money to support such research. I met with a lot of slammed doors, laughter, and frustration. My next step was to turn to media representatives. I thought if I could get them interested, the other pieces would fall into place. But I was wrong.

No one in the media would talk to me. In spite of the fact that the research into angiogenesis had been going on for more

•than twenty years, the people in television and radio thought I was a nut when I broached the topic of shark cartilage as a possible cancer treatment. I tried putting my information together in book form in the hopes of having it published. Every publishing company I approached put me on hold. It seemed as though nothing would ever gel.

Then I phoned Dr. Morton Walker, a professional medical journalist and author. He suggested that I talk to Rudy Shur, managing editor of Avery Publishing Group. I called Rudy who asked me a number of questions in an attempt to ascertain if I was aboveboard. At the end of the conversation, Rudy asked me to send him my manuscript along with the original Harvard and MIT studies on which my work was based. Upon reading the material, he said, "If this stuff is for real, it's probably the most important discovery in the past hundred years toward finding an effective treatment for cancer. However, your manuscript needs a lot of work." Rudy suggested that I work with a writer he knew who had lost several friends and relatives to cancer and whose husband had been doing cancer research for almost twenty years. Eight months later, *Sharks Don't Get Cancer* was published.

When the book first came out, bookstores were reluctant to carry it. Luckily, we found an arm of distribution in health food stores that had book sections. As we tried to get the ball rolling, we found that few newspapers, radio shows, or TV shows were willing to have me talk about shark cartilage. I was fortunate, however, to have a friend who was able to contact Steve Shepherd, an associate producer at *60 Minutes*. Steve expressed interest in reading the book, and found his interest further piqued by the material. The public relations people at Avery; Jonathan Braun, a friend and public relations specialist; my co-author; and I had several conversations with Steve before he submitted his suggestions to the "powers that be" at *60 Minutes*.

Three months later, we heard from the producers of the

show. They were interested in having preliminary discussions about the possibility of doing a segment on shark cartilage. The timing was perfect because I had just gotten the Cuban government's okay to conduct clinical trials in that country. I was very excited, as I'm sure you can imagine, but I was nervous, too. The environment of derision and apathy in which I found myself made me wonder how a program could present me or my work in a positive light. I fully expected the program to rake those involved in the project over the coals. After all, Mike Wallace was known to chop off people's heads, and I was warned that he could make me look like a fool.

Mike Wallace is definitely an up-front guy. Our conversations were actually very pleasant, but I could not know until the show aired whether or not I would be ripped apart. As it turned out, *60 Minutes* was interested in only one thing—the truth. And those involved with the show pursued the facts with "due diligence" like no peer-review journal ever does (someone even called Cornell to see if I had really graduated). *60 Minutes* decided to go all out to determine if shark cartilage actually had therapeutic possibilities. After all, this was cancer, a life-or-death issue.

And so began the discussions preliminary to the shooting. CBS and *60 Minutes* had a protocol about as demanding as any the FDA ever devised. Dedicated to a standard of excellence, this program airs important stories—stories that capture the imagination of the viewer and are timely and interesting. But a TV program truly lives in a glass bowl: Being caught in one false move can be devastating. It means a loss of credibility and possibly the end of the show. Seven years earlier there had been a *60 Minutes* segment on the benefits of laetrile. The show was nailed by the press, by government agencies, and by the scientific community for doing a disservice to the public. From that point on, *60 Minutes* had shied away from stories on any treatment that was alternative in nature. (The show did, however, run one or two segments on interferons and interleukins, potential cancer-treatment breakthroughs developed by main-stream researchers.) As a general rule, however, anything from outside the medical establishment was verboten on *60 Minutes*. This is a number one show; why would they put that reputation in jeopardy?

Finally, after much investigation and deliberation, CBS decided to go ahead with the shark cartilage story. The show's reputation was put on the line. The station and the show were taking a chance on me. CBS was making a substantial investment of time, personnel, and money. Many thousands of dollars were spent to produce a twelve-minute segment. People affiliated with the show accompanied me to Cuba four times. The crew shot many hours of film during different stages of the clinical trial. Mike Wallace himself visited Cuba at the end of the study.

In this study, twenty-nine terminal cancer patients, all of whom had tumor-based cancers and all of whom were classified as either Stage III or Stage IV (the final, most advanced cancer stages), were selected to receive shark cartilage. Most of these patients had previously undergone conventional treatments without success, but none had received any treatment for the five- or six-week period before the study started. All were admitted to a fully staffed clinic to facilitate extensive laboratory testing and record keeping. (See details of study beginning on page 95.)

At the onset of the study, the patients were close to death, flat on their backs. When the TV crew arrived six weeks later, the patients were showing signs of improvement. At the end of twelve weeks, many of the patients were largely well, on their way to recovery. At sixteen weeks, when much of the segment was filmed, many of the patients were much improved.

The consensus of the physicians was unanimous—even if the shark cartilage had not cured the patients, it had "dramatically improved their quality of life." A dramatic demonstration of this improved quality was seen by viewers of *60 Minutes*; Mike Wallace was filmed running alongside an eighty-two-year-old man who, at the onset of the study, was an advanced prostate cancer patient who could not even get out of bed.

This is the story that *60 Minutes* aired, and I couldn't have asked for a more objective report. Gail Eisen, a *60 Minutes* producer, is quoted as saying, "We heard the very impressive presentations of the Cuban doctors. And we could see with our own eyes that some of the tumors were shrinking." She pointed to the case of one woman who had an ovarian tumor the size of a basketball. On the crew's second visit, Eisen said, "We could see that it [the tumor] had markedly diminished. When we see something with our own eyes, it's hard to dismiss it as nothing more than 'anecdotal evidence.'"

The segment was presented as it should have been; it was fair and unbiased. And then six months later, CBS reprised the episode with an update reporting that of the twenty-nine subjects who had participated in the trial, fourteen were still alive and well. As it turned out, if you have an honest story, *60 Minutes* is not "out to get you."

As soon as the bookstores heard that *60 Minutes* was about to air the segment, orders poured in. You could walk into any major bookstore and find ten or twelve copies of *Sharks Don't Get Cancer* on the shelves. But the day after the piece aired, my publisher received only two queries from the media: one from a small Midwestern paper and another from a British journalist operating out of the office of the *Miami Herald*. Although representatives from the media let the issue pass them by, on the day after the broadcast, hundreds of TV viewers—the people who might benefit—contacted CBS, the National Institutes of Health (NIH), and various Congressional offices to ask why I had been forced to conduct clinical trials in Cuba rather than in the United States. And the books began to sell.

For the next six months, stories ran intermittently in United States papers. Some were reasonable and accurate reports of what was going on. Others reported the information in a negative or skeptical manner.

Once my book began getting exposure, I found myself faced with negative press almost daily. On Sunday, May 9, 1993, for instance, the front page of the *Dayton Daily News* in Ohio reported, "Furor over the possible medicinal value of shark cartilage began last year when Dr. I. William Lane of Milburn, N.J., and a co-author, writer Linda Comac, published a book, *Sharks Don't Get Cancer: How Shark Cartilage Could Save Your Life.*" Other articles in magazines, newspapers, and other publications referred to us as "quacks, charlatans, and greedy entrepreneurs." That is, if they referred to us at all.

Mention of the work done by the various physicians and researchers with whom I have been associated was glaringly absent from a front-page report in *The New York Times* in December 1994: "Scientists Report Finding A Way to Shrink Tumors." The article reported the findings of Dr. David Cheresh and Dr. Peter Brooks of the Scripps Research Institute in San Diego, who had announced that in animal experiments (experiments financed by a large grant from the National Institutes of Health) they had discovered a way of making tumors regress with an injection of either of two proteins (see page 113). The article explains that the findings are the result of research into tumor angiogenesis. Previous angiogenesis research had indicated that halting the development of blood vessels would stop tumor growth. "But until the Scripps report, no one had thought that you could get tumor regression," Dr. Judah Folkman is quoted as saying. It is truly astounding that I, the Cuban physicians, other researchers associated with me, the 170 thousand people who have bought *Sharks Don't Get Cancer*, and the estimated 105 million who saw the episode on *60 Minutes* could be construed as "no one." Obviously, Dr. Folkman, a prime example of establishment research, and the reporter from *The New York Times*, the prime voice of the establishment, would never dream of mentioning advocates of alternative medicine or studies involving a natural product. In fact, the *Times* has never run an article on shark cartilage, but reported the study at Scripps

Institute; and in late March 1995, reported that a substance derived from birch bark had been shown to shrink melanomas in mice.

Another notable omission from the various publications is a review of the book. Not one single mainstream publication has reviewed *Sharks Don't Get Cancer* despite the fact that it has sold more than 170 thousand copies, been translated into more than a dozen different languages, and been recognized as a bestseller in the health field.

A few months after the release of *Sharks Don't Get Cancer*, *Publisher's Weekly*, the bible of the publishing industry, noted that the book "has been all but ignored by the mainstream press." Indeed, despite the aggressive attempts of the publisher to interest mainstream media, five hundred advance copies to newspapers and magazines netted only three return calls. *Publisher's Weekly* quotes the publisher as saying, "There is a form of censorship going on in the mainstream media."

Although mainstreamers have yet to review the book, scores of local papers and a host of alternative health magazines have covered the book and the story of shark cartilage from the point of view of its life-saving potential. One of the earliest of these articles appeared in a British publication *The Immortalist* in March 1993. In that same month *Natural Foods Merchandiser* noted of the book, "There has been little press coverage or public discussion.

Press coverage did begin to pick up when I began touring the country with the two physicians who had run the Cuban trials. We visited seven major hospitals in the United States and Canada to present our evidence that shark cartilage is an efficacious cancer therapy. Though meager, the evidence was thorough and included histological slides of cancer tissue before, during, and after whole shark cartilage treatment (see pages 104–106 for some samples of these slides). We spoke to members of the established medical community in hospitals and medical schools because I wanted to get to the physicians who are the first line of attack against cancer. I wanted them to be fully apprised of what was happening in the field.

As we went from city to city, I did lots of radio talk shows. I spoke on the air in California, Boston, Philadelphia, and upstate New York. Following this tour, I went to Australia. What a reception I got there! Not only did I appear on the major talk shows, but every major paper ran a story on the shark cartilage findings. The same thing happened when I went to England. This was completely opposite to the American response. Is it possible that these countries are more open-minded in accepting something outside the mainstream? Apparently, it is.

IN CONCLUSION

Much has been written and said about the power of the mass media in the United States. I think that the coverage received by shark cartilage is an excellent example of just how influential the media is. There's no doubt in my mind that the *60 Minutes* segment spawned an ever-growing amount of interest. As month followed month, network followed network until every major network had aired some report on shark cartilage.

We should not, however, forget that when I first started working with shark cartilage, no one in the media would talk to me. It was actually the power of the written word—the power of *Sharks Don't Get Cancer* to get its message to the people, to the man on the street and to the people affiliated with *60 Minutes*—that got things moving for shark cartilage. Perhaps the combined power of the book and the press helped convince the Food and Drug Administration to approve human trials for shark cartilage. I don't know. I do know that with the media attention I've gotten, it's become easier to make contact with government agencies and talk to important people, trying to ensure that the issue of shark cartilage's efficacy is finally resolved.

4.

The Government
and Me

A Christmas present for the American people.

—President Richard Nixon
announcing the "War on Cancer"
1971

A quarter century ago, former President Richard Nixon declared the "War on Cancer." Since then, billions of dollars have been spent on research, but surgery, radiation, and chemotherapy—scar, burn, and poison—remain the major weapons in a battle we have still not won. The battle plans in this war are not being drawn up at the Pentagon but at the National Cancer Institute (NCI), a division of the National Institutes of Health (NIH), and at the Food and Drug Administration (FDA). These government agencies are fraught with the bureaucratic, political, and budgetary problems traditionally associated with big government and are, in addition, plagued by tunnel vision. The insistence on working with forms of cancer treatment that, at best, do not work, and, at worst, maim or kill has fomented its own war. Many advocates of alternative medical practices are now waging war against the cancer establishment. It is a war in which I have become a tried and tested foot soldier, storming the bulwarks of the NCI and the FDA.

THE FOOD AND DRUG ADMINISTRATION

Every day, scores of people walk into their local pharmacies and buy such products as pain relievers, decongestants, and cough suppressants. Scores more are there to fill prescriptions for blood-pressure medications, insulin, and antibiotics. They plunk down their money, go home with their packages, and expect to see at least *some* results sometime soon. The fulfillment of their expectations rests in large measure with the Food and Drug Administration.

In existence since 1931, the FDA consists of bureaus of food, product safety, drugs, and veterinary medicine. Its job is to protect the nation's health by ensuring that foods and cosmetics are safe, drugs are effective, and products are honestly labeled and packaged. Because of its activities, the FDA has a lot of say in the final verdict on shark cartilage's efficacy as a cancer treatment and/or preventive. I have directed a great deal of time and energy toward that agency.

The FDA will license only those drugs that have been proven safe and effective for the treatment of a particular disease or condition. Federal law defines "drug" as any substance that alters the structure or function of the body. Because government agencies have yet to be convinced that shark cartilage has such an effect on the body, the cartilage presently is being sold as a nutritional supplement, not a drug. The stores in which shark cartilage is sold cannot, therefore, promote it as a cancer therapy. If medicinal claims are made for shark cartilage, retailers risk provoking the wrath of the FDA. If such claims were made, the FDA fraud unit would come into the picture and have the products—of which there are many—removed from the store's shelves.

Natural foods retailers might possibly have trouble on their hands if they sell a product that is not considered a drug along with magazines touting the medical benefits of that product. Even a reprint of an article constitutes a health claim if it's distributed with the product. Those of you who bought this book in a health food store may fear that you are involved in something nefarious. Be aware that the FDA does not consider books or magazines advertisements for a product unless they are placed directly beside that product in a store. In such a case, the FDA can confiscate the product and the literature and possibly jail the seller.

Early in my work, I often worried that the FDA would act precipitously and take action against me, shark cartilage, and even my book. In light of the FDA's long "anti" alternative medicine history, a healthy dosage of justified paranoia was definitely in order. I knew that the agency had invoked its powers of seizure, criminal prosecution, and injunction (halting interstate commerce) numerous times against many pioneers in the field of alternative medicine. It is no wonder that I was once apprehensive of the FDA.

To my surprise, this powerful watchdog agency has not been a roadblock; rather, it has been something of a white knight. I have found that all of my dealings with the FDA have been highly professional and quite pleasant. I have come to truly appreciate the work of the agency regarding my situation and the receptive attitude of Dr. Gregory Burke, past head of New Drug Evaluation at FDA. As it turned out, it was FDA representatives who literally forced NIH to include shark cartilage in its data bank of cancer treatments.

Actually, FDA investigators did come to my office once because they had heard I was selling shark cartilage and the book *Sharks Don't Get Cancer* as well as disseminating a shark cartilage newsletter. What they saw was exactly what anyone would expect at the office of a consultant—heaps of disheveled papers; an overworked assistant (Norma); and me, on the phone. Satisfied that I was not running a shark cartilage super-market, they doffed their caps—at least figuratively—and left. Then at the pre-IND (investigational new drug) meeting, I was asked, "How can we help you? All we want to know is the truth. Help prove to us that it is effective." That's all I've ever wanted to do, and now that two different shark cartilage products have IND status, the proof is at hand.

Investigational New Drug (IND) Status

With the awarding of the first full-fledged IND for shark carti-lage by the FDA in November 1994, the cartilage became an experimental therapy, a "new product under investigation." This IND can lead to approval of shark cartilage as a drug while it is still available as a food supplement.

A drug is considered investigational if it is a molecular entity that is not in the marketplace, or is a recognized sub-stance that will be used in a new way, in a new combination, or for a new clinical indication. In brief, an untested use for any established substance is an investigational use. (For this reason, practitioners of alternative medicine or ethnomedicine often feel their agents are not investigational new drugs and do not even apply for INDs.)

An IND application must be filed if an "investigational drug" is to be administered to humans or, if it is a veterinary drug, to animals. Basically, investigational new drug status is an exemption from the laws governing marketed drugs. One of the items required in an IND application is a protocol or plan of action. If the protocol includes human subjects, the investi-gator must secure the approval of an institutional review board (IRB), a board comprised of professionals who decide whether the studies can be conducted at their institutions.

The FDA does not itself test products. Investigational new drugs are tested in highly regulated and controlled studies called clinical trials. These trials follow a concrete plan that not only answers various questions, but must safeguard the subjects or patients. Patients can become involved in the clinical trial only if their medical conditions meet the specifics outlined in the IND protocol.

The road to drug licensure by the FDA normally consists of four phases. Phase I determines the safety of the drug or device, usually with animal subjects. In Phase II, which usually involves studying the drug in numerous patients during clinical trials, efficacy is established. During Phase III, researchers determine appropriate dosage and try to ascertain long-term effects. They also compare the investigational treatment with standard treatments and evaluate which is better. Phase IV establishes the investigational treatment as a standard therapy.

A drug's journey through all the phases of clinical trials—from its discovery to its licensing by the FDA—can take an average of twelve years and cost about $360 million. The cost is normally borne by the company that wishes to market the drug. This company usually contracts with a research institution, which will find the subjects, monitor them, and provide the data. Only one of every five drugs that goes through this involved procedure typically makes it to market. (On an international basis, it is estimated that pharmaceutical companies synthesize 6,200 compounds for every one that is approved.)

Over the past several years, there has been pressure to update the whole drug review situation. Drug companies want speed so they can get a better return on their investment. Those who are ill and their loved ones want life-saving medications to be available before it's too late. The FDA has, therefore, developed several more expeditious systems (see *Speeding the Drug Review Process* beginning on page 50). In 1992, consider that 387 new drugs and biological products were submitted for FDA review. Of these, 91 eventually received approval with a

Speeding the Drug Review Process

It costs millions and takes years for a new drug to earn approval from the Food and Drug Administration. Until all the data are in and the drug is approved, the people who need the medication must do without—sometimes die without. Since the late 1980s, the FDA has made a concentrated effort to speedily get new drugs to those who need them.

Treatment INDs (investigational new drugs) were created so that certain experimental agents could be used to treat seriously ill patients. Normally, an IND is granted when an agent is being investigated to gain information about its safety and effectiveness. In other words, treatment INDs make certain experimental drugs available to patients before those drugs receive final FDA approval.

With treatment INDs, the burden of proof is on the manufacturer, who must show the FDA that the drug in question is safe and effective. The product's sponsor—a pharmaceutical company, private organization, government agency, or individual— must show scientific evidence that the product may work. Results of the trials are submitted to the FDA for determination of whether benefits outweigh risks. Reviews of products for the most life-threatening diseases can be completed in less than a year.

During the review process, the FDA provides labeling inserts, which are given to physicians along with the products that have gotten treatment INDs. These inserts provide the physicians with the information they need to prescribe the drug safely at appropriate doses.

Treatment INDs allow drug developers to provide earlier and wider access to promising investigational therapies for patients with special or immediately life-threatening diseases for which there is no other treatment. The protocol for a treatment IND spells out the criteria for special or life-threatening conditions. Sponsors are informed what scientific information about the drug's safety and potential usefulness must be on hand, and physicians are told how to obtain the investigational drugs for treatment use. This type of IND does not lead to drug classification down the line; clinical trials will still be required. Furthermore, treatment INDs provide for very limited use of the drug.

A treatment IND, like a clinical trial, requires "informed patient consent." Participating subjects must be fully informed of the protocol and possible side effects of the drug, and they must freely give their consent after receiving the information. The FDA stipulates that during the trials, the product cannot be promoted or otherwise commercialized. A product administered under a treatment IND must currently be undergoing or must have completed active clinical investigation, and its sponsor must be pursuing marketing approval with "due diligence."

By January 1993, twenty-eight agents had been granted treatment IND status. By October 1993, twenty-two of these were available in the marketplace. Treatment INDs became well-known because of their role in AIDS; a treatment IND expanded the availability of AZT (Zidovudine) for people suffering from this disease. Testing of thirty-three patients in 1985 led to a Phase II trial to assess the safety and effectiveness of AZT. The trial began in February 1986 and involved 300 patients. In September 1986, a treatment protocol was written and 4,000 people were treated even before the drug received approval.

Another fast-track procedure allows limited use of experimental medicines while they are still being tested. "Compassionate use" permits sponsors of investigational agents to provide those agents to physicians. The doctors cannot be involved in the controlled clinical trials of the agents but may use them for individual patients who might be helped.

In its efforts to get medications to those who need them, the FDA has instituted an IND category that refers to "priority drugs." For these, the FDA and the drug's sponsor work together at the earliest stage of investigation. Studies are planned to ensure that all of the information necessary for a decision will be on hand as soon as possible. When the marketing application for a priority drug is submitted, the FDA mobilizes to review the application and render its decision as quickly as possible.

To further expedite the delivery of effective treatment to the public, the FDA turned its attention to cutting costs. The Prescription Drug User Fee Act of 1992 permits the FDA to collect user fees from product developers to cover the cost of expediting review of prescription drug applications. In this way, the FDA does not have to rely entirely on tax dollars. Cutting the costs and time involved in getting drugs to the marketplace is of great value to the consumer.

median review time of 22.6 months; 4 were reviewed in less than 8 months: Hivid for treating advanced HIV, Halfan for malaria, Nepron for *pneumocystis carnii*, and Taxol for ovarian cancer.

We must remember that the FDA needs to strike a balance between helping and safeguarding the public while permitting scientific inquiry. In reviewing an IND application, FDA evaluates the risks and benefits to the subjects in the trial. People at the FDA were so impressed by the preliminary results of shark cartilage research that they agreed to bypass animal studies and award an IND for Phase II human testing. This means the FDA has agreed that shark cartilage is nontoxic; that's a given. Generally, research to prove a substance is not toxic can last for five years and cost millions of dollars. At the pre-IND meetings, I was told, "We heard it works—just prove to us that it works and we promise you a quick acceptance." Those were the words I had worked eight years to hear: "Just prove it to us." Perhaps it is fortuitous that government agencies did not get into the act initially. We'd have spent years doing animal studies before being permitted to work with humans. To my knowledge, this is the first time that a whole natural product has ever been approved for full human Phase II trials. In fact, the FDA has approved only one health claim for a food supplement: Extra calcium may help protect the elderly against osteoporosis.

The clinical trials now being conducted will investigate and, hopefully, establish the safety and efficacy of shark cartilage for a specific clinical use. The requirements for a clinical trial conducted under an IND are:

- Clinical protocol must be approved by an institutional review board (IRB).
- Subjects must give informed consent of their own free will.
- Identities of the subjects are protected.
- The substance being tested must be produced or prepared so as to ensure quality, stability, consistency, and potency.
- Subjects may leave the clinical trial at any time.
- All records and information are maintained and available for inspection.
- Investigators are required to show respect for the subjects— assure privacy and confidentiality; get informed consent; and protect children, pregnant women, prisoners, and others with "diminished autonomy."
- If they know the consequences of the substance being tested, investigators must not use it in a way that will harm subjects. If they are unsure of the consequences, they must do everything possible to maximize the benefits and minimize the harm.

These requirements, now known as the Belmont Report, were first laid down in the 1976 National Commission for the Protection of Human Subjects of Biomedical and Behavioral Research and are now in the Code of Federal Regulations. Any institution applying to receive federal funding for research must agree to these regulations. That institution assures NIH's Office of Protection from Research Risks of its compliance, and files a document called an assurance. Part of the assurance is the commitment to establish an institutional review board. Members of the IRB are carefully chosen by the group running the trials.

Among government officials and people involved in medical research, the consensus seems to be that those who promote questionable treatments rarely submit information to FDA about their products, let alone reliable and accurate data. Obviously, shark cartilage passed out of the realm of "questionable treatments" as soon as application for an IND was made. Granting of the IND moves shark cartilage into the spot once occupied by such new drugs as Taxol, AZT, and interleukin—potentially into the realm of mainstream medicine. The IND status should force mainstream investigators to consider shark cartilage a "respectable" substance even if they previously had doubts.

THE NATIONAL CANCER INSTITUTE

Even though the FDA is taking shark cartilage's potential seriously, other government agencies have been more difficult. In my last book, I briefly discussed my up-and-down relationship with the National Cancer Institute (NCI), a federal agency that conducts and supports biomedical research into the causes, cure, and prevention of cancer.

At first, NCI wanted nothing to do with me. However, when I addressed Robert Gallo, M.D., chief of the Laboratory of Tumor Cell Biology, and other investigators from the institute, I received a standing ovation and was promised that studies using shark cartilage in the treatment of Kaposi's sarcoma (KS) would soon begin. I was assured that NCI's people would work in coordination with me, sharing their results. Just three months later, I was told shark cartilage research would not be pursued because NCI doesn't deal in the "cures," but in the "mechanisms" of cancer. NCI representatives also felt that it would "serve" my own interests if the organization appeared to be interested in shark cartilage. No longer was the issue seen as an inquiry into whether shark cartilage worked, whether it could save lives.

Subsequently, I heard that NCI was being very negative about my work so I decided to check on it. Without identifying myself, I called the agency, asking for information about shark cartilage. I was transferred to the person "responsible" for disseminating that information. When he recommended that I speak to a physician in New Jersey, I asked, "What about talking to Dr. Lane?"

"Don't bother; the guy's a charlatan," was the abrupt response. A bureaucrat whom I had never met, who had never asked for any information, was telling me that what I was doing was not legitimate.

I spoke to my co-author and told her what was occurring. She also called the institute, was referred to the same person for information about shark cartilage, and was told the same thing I had been told. The word from NCI was, indeed, negative, and was being passed without any information behind it.

NCI calls me a "fraud" and does not recommend shark cartilage for cancer patients even though the *Journal of the National Cancer Institute* says, "Most researchers agree that continued study of the shark's intriguing anatomy may yield answers to treating cancer in humans."

The possibility that NCI is not willing to seriously consider alternative medical therapies is no secret. Various members of Congress had been lobbying for an organization that would investigate such therapies in an effort to find the truth. In January 1993, Congress formed the Office of Alternative Medicine (OAM), which is a branch of the NCI. Joseph Jacobs, M.D., was chosen to head this office.

Dr. Jacob's first task was to go through numerous proposals and select those treatments to be studied. From the outset, he informed several people that shark cartilage would be one of the treatments investigated. On Monday, August 2, 1993, the *Wall Street Journal* reported that OAM would study various alternative treatments: "After a slow start, the NIH office now is getting down to work. It will analyze the benefits of attacking cancer through Dr. Revichi's treatments [biological guided chemotherapy including coffee enemas], and will assess the cancer-fighting characteristics of shark cartilage and one other anticancer treatment. . . . The program will fund preliminary studies of 20 other unconventional cures."

Months later, NIH had changed its mind. Dr. Jacobs said he would rather support research aimed at isolating an active ingredient in cartilage. Work, he pointed out, that was already ongoing at NIH.

In elucidating the turnaround, NIH spokesman Mark Stern said, "The previous data [on shark cartilage therapy] does not merit further investigation. It doesn't work. It's costing people a lot of money, time, and hopes. It's not worth it." Stern also said, "It is very difficult for a patient to achieve a therapeutic dose." He explained that this is, at least in part, because the proteins in the cartilage are not well absorbed. The issue of absorption, however, is far from resolved. Much scientific data indicates that proteins may indeed be absorbed intact (see pages 158–163). Furthermore, cancer patients who are currently taking shark cartilage often report that they begin to feel better after four weeks; in six weeks, pain frequently diminishes; in eight weeks, tumors may begin to shrink. These people don't seem to be having trouble "achieving" a "therapeutic dose." In any event, Stern's words imply that there *is* a therapeutic dose—he just claims it's very high.

Perhaps the most pressing question raised by Stern is the issue of "worth." How can anyone wonder whether the effort is "worth" it, or whether the chance of saving thousands of lives a year is "worth" a piece of NIH's $1.9 billion annual cancer research expenditure? Consider that Kyl Green, director of managed care at the Health Insurance Association of America, says that insurers like alternative medicines that can be used to prevent disease and avoid surgery; costs are kept low. One-third of Americans use alternative treatments, and insurance companies are increasingly willing to pay because the treatments are less expensive than conventional ones. Isn't the curbing of medical costs a major issue in the political arena? Furthermore, how can NIH dismiss shark cartilage because "it doesn't work" when the Office of Alternative Medicine was established to determine *if* the various alternative therapies in which people are investing time, money, and hopes actually do work.

Interestingly, Dr. Jacobs himself seems to have had difficulty answering that question. In the July 15, 1994, issue of *Science*, it was reported Dr. Jacobs would be resigning his position as of September. According to the magazine, "Outsiders say that Jacobs ran afoul of the activists who lobbied to create the alternative medicine program. . . . They wanted Jacobs to devote more time and money to investigating controversial therapies—such as the use of shark cartilage to treat cancer and arthritis." Wayne B. Jonas, M.D., replaced Dr. Jacobs and is the current head of the OAM. Dr. Jonas is an outstanding director whose open-minded approach to alternative medicine offers hope in the research and development of such treatments.

Frank Wiewel, founder of People Against Cancer in Otho, Iowa, says, "There is good evidence, not proof mind you, that shark cartilage may be effective in preventing cancer." Yet, NIH claims "previous data does not merit further investigation." Previous data includes the results of the clinical studies in Cuba, in which approximately 50 percent of the patients had significant improvement in their conditions. Consider that the response rate for interleukin-2 was reported in the October 5, 1990, issue of *Science* to be 18 to 20 percent. One oncologist was quoted as saying, "I've never seen anything like the response rate we get with IL-2."

Speaking for the National Institutes of Health, Mark Stern says the issue would be reconsidered if new scientific evidence came to light and it satisfied NIH. Perhaps that evidence will come from NIH itself. It has been reported that NCI scientists as well as researchers at MIT are still working to isolate a substance in shark cartilage that may halt the spread of cancer. These very scientists and researchers who pursue their own avenues of research—usually with government funding or tax-free foundation grants—have been among my noisiest critics. They never consider that I funded much of the early shark cartilage research out of my own pocket.

My encounters with official apathy have been frustrating and frightening, but I often wonder whether that apathy is something more. Sometimes I think it's a case of "methinks the lady doth protest too much." Do these investigators have vested interests that they do not wish to have upset?

The initals NIH are sometimes known to stand for "not invented here." We're dealing with egos, and perhaps NIH people won't pay attention to work done outside the agency. I have the same misgivings about NCI, a branch of NIH.

As I mentioned earlier, during my initial dealings with NIH, I met with Robert Gallo, M.D., chief of the Laboratory of Tumor Cell Biology at NCI. I have found Dr. Gallo to be one of the most open-minded, brightest, and supportive people at NIH. He is the only one in that organization who spoke to me after the *60 Minutes* story aired, and he was most encouraging.

Dr. Gallo had originally agreed to do studies using shark cartilage on Kaposi's sarcoma (KS), a cancer that commonly develops in AIDS patients. The studies were later cancelled. Interestingly, Dr. Gallo is co-author of an article about a patented drug that inhibits angiogenesis. The article, which appeared in the March 13, 1992, issue of *Science*, details the research on Kaposi's sarcoma in rats conducted by Dr. Gallo and scientists from a Japanese pharmaceutical company. The drug being used was found to inhibit blood vessel proliferation in rat KS. Are we looking at a conflict of interest or is it just that stall tactics are part and parcel of bureaucracy? Some of you may recall that when the War on Cancer was declared by President Nixon in the early 1970s, it was believed that an all-out battle could not be waged by NCI because work would be stifled by layers of HEW (Department of Health, Education, and Welfare) bureaucracy. Isn't it ironic that one of the recently approved FDA trials for shark cartilage involves subjects with advanced cases of nonresponsive Kaposi's sarcoma? If the NIH had done the study on KS when they had originally agreed to, we would be that much further ahead of the game now.

Perhaps even more detrimental to research than bureaucracy is the "old-boy network" or system of peer review. It is a system that has long been suspect. If we look again at the early days of the War on Cancer, we will note that when William Ballenger was named an assistant to the secretary of HEW, one of his jobs was to facilitate the review process for grants. The two-step process involves a peer review in which "peer experts" look at the scientific merit of a proposed project. Next, the grant application is reviewed by advisory councils comprised of nongovernment scientists and laymen (who turn down about 5 percent of the grants recommended by the peer review). Members of the councils know the needs and resources of their fields, but there has often been skepticism about the process' efficiency. It has also been suggested that the review process has an "ingrown incestuous pork barrel quality." Consider that when Mr. Ballenger sought to fill several vacancies on these councils in 1975, he eliminated those candidates who believed that NIHers made up an "old-boy network."

As recently as August 1994, *Science* reported, "Federal research agencies have long been thought to shelter 'old-boy networks' and to favor insiders who know the system." The General Accounting Office (GAO), Congress's investigative branch, looked into the allegations as requested by Senator John Glenn (D-Ohio), past chairman of the Senate Governmental Affairs Committee. GAO focused its study on the National Institutes of Health, the National Science Foundation (NSF), and the National Endowment for the Humanities (NEH). It then released a 133-page report, which includes findings of "empirical evidence of potential problems." GAO found that at NSF, familiarity with an applicant was correlated to better scores, and that at all three agencies, there was a lack of explicit criteria for judging proposals.

IN CONCLUSION

I think it is only a matter of time before shark cartilage becomes a recognized weapon in the war against cancer. Shark cartilage advocates have presented the evidence garnered thus far. In light of those facts, FDA has decided shark cartilage is nontoxic and should be evaluated during controlled clinical trials. If those trials are successful, shark cartilage will, hopefully, be included among the treatments that NIH refers to as "state of the art." Once government agencies are on our side, so to speak, the scientific establishment is almost certain to follow.

5.

The Scientific Community Reacts

Why the insistence on present modes of treatment that plainly do not work? Why the refusal to investigate new possibilities? Why is there this refusal on the part of this money-hungry industry, this industry that is itself something of a malignant growth? ... Even if a cure for cancer were found, it would pay them to hide or destroy such a cure. It would be good business to do so.

—Keith Alan Lasko, M.D.
The Great Billion Dollar Medical Swindle

As we have seen, the leading players in the scientific establishment dealing with cancer are government agencies: the National Cancer Institute (NCI) and the Food and Drug Administration (FDA). Between the huge budgets at their command and the political clout they wield, their operations set the tone for the entire scientific establishment. No scientist wants to buck these agencies. If a scientist did so, he or she would literally put his or her livelihood at risk. The scientist's reputation would be severely impugned and chances of receiving funding for research would be nil. "Getting a piece of the action" has never been easy for those who are outside the scientific establishment. As a proponent of shark cartilage, I have fared no better. Established researchers, many of whom have been funded by or hope to be funded by NCI, scoff at my work. They misquote or ignore me, take material out of context, and stoop to name-calling. In short, they resort to every time-honored propaganda technique. Could Dr. Lasko be right in his belief that cancer researchers, physicians, foundation executives, etc. are more interested in keeping their jobs than in curing cancer?

It's interesting to note that the original hypothesis indicating that tumor growth could be arrested by halting development of new blood vessels was considered heresy by the establishment. Dr. Folkman, who developed the hypothesis, says that to this day, no one has ever requested a reprint of the paper in which he presented the concept. Even before Folkman's paper, as early as 1939 and again in 1945, research papers discuss the role of vascularization in cancer. These issues were largely ignored by a medical establishment dominated by the surgeon.

I can't help but wonder if some of the criticisms leveled against me are motivated by the wish of scientists to dominate the field. Or are many scientists so set in their beliefs that they cannot recognize even the possibility that a whole natural product can be an effective therapeutic agent?

Mainstream researchers and physicians have long fought against the use of natural substances. According to William Stetler-Stevenson, M.D., Ph.D., of NCI's Laboratory of Pathology, "As medical scientists, our training and approach has been to emphasize 'rational drug design.' This means that first we try to develop some understanding of how or why a drug works. We can then begin to modify the drug with the specific aim of improving upon the therapeutic effectiveness of the parent compound." That's all well and better than good, but why think about modifying for the purposes of improving *before* you even have the drug? Why not work *with* the substance, modifying and improving it as you go along?

Even Dr. Langer who has already demonstrated that an extract of shark cartilage is an effective inhibitor of angiogenesis in rabbit corneas (see page 9) speaks of isolating the molecule in cartilage that acts as an angiogenesis inhibitor. The next step in the rational drug design plan would be to produce those molecules in the laboratory. This would be a wonderful event that might eventually lower the cost of shark cartilage as well as protect the shark population. However, the purified chemical is often more costly for many reasons including research expenses and large profit margins. In the meantime, in the United States alone, 600 thousand people per year—not statistics but people—fathers, mothers, children—are dying. Must they wait for the laboratory when an alternative is available?

It is true that my research into shark cartilage's potential as a cancer treatment has been conducted in the field—with people—rather than in the laboratory with test tubes and computers. Do research scientists reject my work because they are so enamored of the sterile laboratory setting that they have forgotten the needs of the people? Or do they want all cancer research conducted in laboratories so that a certain few can maintain control?

Perhaps in an attempt to maintain control, the science industry is dominated by the concept of peer review. Grants are made based upon peer review, and articles are published in certain journals through the same system. Although the system is suspect, as seen in *Peer Review Misses the Mark* beginning on page 64, my lack of publications in "peer-review journals" is one of the major criticisms leveled against me by the mainstream scientific community.

THE ABSORPTION ISSUE

The issue of the body's ability to absorb the active proteins in shark cartilage is the most scientifically valid question raised

Peer Review Misses the Mark

Trial by a jury of peers is a basic—and cherished—tenet of American democracy, dating back to the common-law system of England. The underlying concept is that one should be judged by equals, not by superiors who may look down at you, nor by those beneath you who may fear or be jealous of you. In a stratified or class society, this is eminently important. But, perhaps, the system works less well in a classless society. Certainly, the system of peer review in scientific circles has been beset by problems.

Can there be any efficacy to peer review in the awarding of grants or the choosing of material to be published? In these areas, politics is certain to come into play and the concept of "one hand washes the other" may be preeminent.

*In the October 1994, issue of **Working Woman**, an epidemiologist at the University of Maryland School of Medicine is quoted as saying that peer reviewers "are more likely to fund a 'name,' or someone from an institution like Harvard, rather than an unknown from a lesser institution with a proposal that may be more promising." Roger Jacobs, Ph.D., director of the surgical research laboratory at Metropolitan Hospital Center in New York City, says, "Heaven help the young scientist. He may be brilliant, his work may be on-the-mark, but the most he can hope for is 'approved but not funded.'" The American Cancer Society's scientific-program director is quoted in **Working Woman** as saying, "We can fund only 10% of new research-grant applications, so we're less willing to fund novel and risky projects, even if they rank in the 'excellent' range, rather than the 'outstanding.'"*

*In light of recent scandals involving scientists of some caliber, peer review cannot help but be suspect. As reported in Long Island's **Newsday** on April 10, 1994, "The methods for tracking and preventing misbehavior—such as expert review of scientific papers before publication are imperfect at best."*

In mid-April 1994, a congressional investigation committee chaired by Representative John Dingell (D-Michigan) convened to answer a multitude of questions regarding scientific misconduct in cancer research. The investigation was motivated in large part by the reports of falsified data in a study of the comparative merits of mastectomies and lumpectomies that changed the way breast cancer is treated. The lumpectomy study, conducted in 1985 by the National Surgical Adjuvant Breast and Bowel Project, showed it isn't necessary to remove the entire breast with early cancers.

The study was led by Bernard Fisher, Ph.D., of the University of Pittsburgh, who has been called "the Pittsburgh eminence" by one newspaper. The highly regarded scientist was approached in 1992 by administrators of the National Cancer Institute, who felt that his system for preventing fraud was not as good as it should be. Fisher's indignation at the suggestion brought an apology from the NCI. It has now been revealed, however, that fraud had indeed existed for thirteen years before it was discovered. Some wonder how detection could have taken so long. A Newsday reporter points to Fisher's "solicitous Washington overseers," who maintained the same relationship with him for two years 'after' the discovery, until Congress threatened action.

The disclosure that has now shaken the medical and scientific community and shattered the public's confidence centers around falsified data. This is not a new problem in scientific circles. You may recall that in the mid-1970s, it was revealed that a researcher at Memorial Sloan-Kettering Cancer Center had been painting rats to simulate clinical evidence.

Consider, too, the case of Tufts University's immunologist Thereza Imanishi-Kari accused of falsifying data in a paper published in Cell about a decade ago. A hearing concerning this matter, conducted by the Department of Health and Human Services, began on June 12, 1995. In November, the department's investigatory branch concluded that the immunologist had "fabricated and falsified" results and had further fabricated data to support the falsified findings. Part of the defense rests on the premise that the scientist's record keeping was sloppy—written on paper towels that had been left to yellow on window sills—rather than falsified. If Dr. Imanishi-Kari is found guilty, she will probably be banned from receiving federal funding for ten years.

In the "lumpectomy" scandal, Dr. Roger Poisson at St. Luc Hospital in Montreal had been submitting falsified data to Dr. Fisher from 1977 to 1990. Dr. Poisson claims the data was falsified in order to allow women who were not eligible for the trial to be able to participate. At the root of the problems that NCI later brought to Fisher's attention is the fact that he was not looking at patients' actual records. He was seeing "copies" of x-rays and lab reports, which are less likely to show signs of alteration.

Reports indicate that after the facts about the falsification became known, Fisher published nine new papers. He submitted an additional seven papers even after NCI ordered him to stop using the data. It should, however, be noted that Dr. Fisher has never been charged with misconduct. In fact, in 1995 he was named the first scientific director of the National Surgical Adjuvant Breast and Bowel Project. Fisher was named to the position by Norman Wolmark, who had succeeded Fisher as chair and principal investigator of the lumpectomy project. In reporting the appointment, Science called Wolmark "Fisher's longtime friend and collaborator." Other members of the scientific community seemed enthusiastic over Fisher's reinstatement. One noted geneticist praised him by saying, "There is nothing more heroic than stubbornness in a good cause."

No matter how one feels about Dr. Fisher, the publicity revolving around him and NCI's inability to prevent or halt fraud raises interesting questions about peer review. The specter of pervasive scientific fraud appears when one considers the results of a recent survey of 2,600 graduate students and faculty published in American Scientist. Six to nine percent of those surveyed reported having direct knowledge of faculty members who had plagiarized or falsified data.

Guarantees about the validity of research have not been left entirely in the hands of the participants. One of the most important checks on fraud has been the traditional requirement that any experimental discovery be duplicated by other laboratories before being accepted as valid. The Food and Drug Administration has required auditing of drug trials since 1977, and the National Cancer Institute has required audit studies since 1982. Most research groups fulfil their obligation by sending an audit team to the site. This may not be enough.

According to one government official quoted in the **Newsday** *article, "Dingell thinks big-time scientists are given too much slack, that no one calls them to account, that big scientists are arrogant and insensitive." Bruce Chabner, director of the cancer treatment branch of NCI, seems to concur when he says, "We should have taken action earlier. . . . We are setting up a system where this is not going to happen again." This system includes auditing of 10 percent of patient charts and mandatory site reviews at least once every three years.*

It seems that scientific publications also need a system of review that will work better than peer review. Dr. Drummond Rennie, deputy editor of the **Journal of the American Medical Association,** *has recommended an audit of data behind a random sample of manuscripts accepted for publication. "The bottom line," says Chabner in the* **Newsday** *article, "is you have to have some quality assurance built in."*

by my critics. People in the medical field repeatedly question the efficacy of the oral administration of shark cartilage. Many scientists doubt that humans can absorb the protein components in an active form. Some say that oral administration of large molecules, such as the active protein in shark cartilage, results in the destruction of the molecules. Some physicians also believe that orally administered proteins will be digested or destroyed before they can be effective against tumors. They point to insulin as a classic example. Indeed, in past years, oral administration of insulin proved ineffective for diabetics. However, recent developments in gastrointestinal research indicate that proteins are getting into the bloodstream in much larger sizes than previously thought (see pages 158–163). By the early 1980s, it was even being reported that in experiments conducted on rats, some orally administered insulin was being absorbed in a biologically active form.

In the December 1993, issue of the *Journal of the National Cancer Institute,* Brian Blackadar, M.D., of the Department of Nutritional Sciences at the University of Guelph in Canada, cites several studies showing that small amounts of dipeptides, tripeptides, and tiny amounts of protein fragments and even of intact proteins have been found in the systemic circulation. In other words, the molecules had passed through the intestine relatively intact. In concluding his review of some of the literature on the subject, Dr. Blackadar points to the need to be skeptical about new cancer therapies but entreats us not to dismiss anyone's work too quickly.

THE ROOT OF ALL EVIL

The same scientists who want me to be cautious like other researchers are quick to reject my work. They say my studies are not scientific, the evidence is anecdotal, and I stand to make a profit. Yet they are often the very scientists who for years refused to participate in studies that could produce the necessary scientific evidence. And criticizing me for making a profit is not the point— the real issue is whether or not shark cartilage works.

Making money is not in and of itself an evil thing. Isn't that what capitalism is all about? Perhaps the problem is that scientists do not traditionally see themselves as players in the capitalist system. Indeed, Americans have long divided scientists into two roles—"pure" and "applied." Pure scientists see money as a pursuit unworthy of a man of intellect. They work only for truth and knowledge, without considering whether their labors might bring financial gain to anyone. On the other hand, those known as applied scientists turn theories and facts into market-able items. Pure scientists have, therefore, always been scornful of applied scientists.

SHARK PRESERVATION

One pure scientist who is often lined up on the opposite side of the fence from me is Carl Luer, Ph.D. One of the foremost shark researchers in the nation, Dr. Luer is a biochemist at Mote Marine Laboratory in Sarasota, Florida. Actually, he and I are very much in agreement.

Dr. Luer is concerned about what he calls "the cartilage frenzy." He fears people may "gulp" shark cartilage pills and not consult physicians. It is true that the attention given to shark cartilage has created something of a frenzy; just consider the copycat products discussed in Chapter 11. But it would be sheer folly for anyone to gulp shark cartilage without consulting a physician. Certainly, anyone who has cancer must be under a doctor's care (see Chapter 10 for information on finding and working with a doctor that is right for you.)

Shark cartilage is not to be viewed as an alternative to tradi-tional therapies. So far, it has been tested only on those for whom conventional therapies have been tried without success. And those who are using shark cartilage for relief from the pain of arthritis should be monitored by a physician in case there is a need for medical intervention. And, finally, those of us involved in shark cartilage research are *hungry* for the data that can be provided by physicians working with arthritis and/or cancer patients. Clinical information about the patient's condition before and after using shark cartilage is vital to our research.

Another of Luer's worries has been that the demand for cartilage will endanger survival of the species, already a depleted population with 215,338 sharks reported caught in 1966 and 370,458 in 1991. Based on the weight of shark fins going into the Orient for shark-fin soup, these figures account for only a fraction of the sharks caught. I am not ignoring the issue. I am fully aware that some species of shark are in danger, and I know full well that people have tended to ignore ecological issues with often heartbreaking results. Ecologically speaking, the shark provides an important balance in nature. As a predator, the shark controls fish overpopulation and removes diseased or injured fish.

There is legitimate concern that sharks are vulnerable to extinction because of their low reproductive capability, long reproductive cycle, and late sexual maturity. Sharks will not breed in captivity, and many do not survive when caught because they simply stop eating. Shark "farming" is, therefore, not viable. According to Sonja Fordham, fishery program specialist with the Center for Marine Conservation, "We must work to conserve what we have. The medicinal value of sharks is another reason we should manage them wisely." According to Ms. Fordham, of the 380 species of shark, three are in danger—the whale shark, the white shark, and the basking shark—and the hammerhead and tiger sharks have had a dramatic decrease in number over the past decade. Ms. Fordham points out that another thirty-nine species of shark require management to protect them. She looks forward to commercial quotas, recreational bag limits, and the requirement of permits—all of which I heartily endorse.

Many fishing experts feel that the federally imposed sanctions against shark fishing in certain areas will adequately protect the species in those areas. More important protection might be afforded sharks by targeting waterfront land developers. These builders fill in and eliminate the wetlands where fish breed, cutting off the supply of fish needed to feed and preserve the sharks who go where the food is. Without wetlands, fish and sharks will both suffer. But I never read about the developers, only about overfishing; this oversight reveals purely economic concerns. And if we do take economics into consideration, there are those who say that when shark fishing is a thriving industry, fishermen themselves will want to protect their livelihood. Simply put, "Why bite the hand that feeds you?"

In contrast, much shark fishing today is purely wasteful—sports enthusiasts seek trophies to hang on their walls; tuna fishermen remove sharks' fins to sell to the Chinese and throw the rest of the dead shark back in the water. A viable shark-fishing industry would certainly curtail the later practice. Indeed, the carcasses would yield sufficient cartilage to make the needed supplements.

Dr. Luer is justifiably concerned about the possible effect of the use of shark cartilage on the worldwide shark population. I, too, am concerned about the possibility of sharks—indeed, of any species—becoming endangered. Remember, I started my career in animal nutrition. I feel strongly, however, that the fears are ill-founded. The crux of the matter is that tons of sharks are being caught and their carcasses tossed back into the sea once their fins have been removed. We can now make excellent use of what had been so criminally wasted. Shark cartilage products can be mass produced using the skulls and spines of fish that have already been killed for their fins.

You may wonder why the cost of shark cartilage food supplements is high if the product utilizes what was once waste. You must remember that the method of cleaning and preparing the cartilage is labor-intensive and, therefore, very costly. The cost is also dependant on the fact that it takes approximately six pounds of frozen cartilage to make one pound of dry shark cartilage powder. Furthermore, fishermen with limited refrigerated holding space at sea will not bring in the heads and backbones unless they receive sufficient economic incentive.

It is my hope that if people come to see the shark as the biological marvel that it is, they may learn to venerate rather than destroy it. All we've learned about ecology and conservation has brought us a long way from the days of the whaling ships.

Then, too, I am not so naive as to believe that shark cartilage will "corner" the market on antiangiogenic agents. There are other such agents already in clinical trials (see page 111–121), and the use of natural shark cartilage may become obsolete before too long. If clinical trials prove its efficacy as a cancer-inhibitor, it will be only a matter of time—and a short time at that—until pharmaceutical companies develop a viable synthetic antiangiogenic agent. Although many people will prefer to use the natural whole shark cartilage, which I believe will be better because it contains a complex blend of effective proteins and mucopolysaccharides, others will, undoubtedly, welcome a synthetic option.

While there may be differences between Carl Luer's point of view and mine, I am glad that his work—which is now getting the recognition it deserves—may one day be instrumental in curing disease. Long interested in sharks' apparent ability to resist cancer, he has spent more than a decade experimenting on sharks and skates (both are fish of the Chondrichthyes class, characterized by a cartilaginous skeleton), injecting them with carcinogens. It is said that he injected some of the "worst substances" into the animals, which still did not develop cancerous tumors in these circumstances. Luer believes there is more than one mechanism involved in sharks' resistance. According to a Gannett News Service reporter, Luer is presently focusing on purifying cartilage molecules and seeking answers to the resistance.

PURIFICATION: BOON OR BANE?

Although Dr. Luer and I agree on several points, we are definitely at a parting of the ways when it comes to the issue of "purifying cartilage molecules." This is actually the major bone of contention between me and most of the establishment researchers.

Believing it virtually impossible to get FDA approval for a pure shark cartilage product, researchers have spent the last twenty years trying to isolate, purify, and then synthesize the protein (or proteins) *in* shark cartilage that is responsible for the antiangiogenic activity—and have done so with limited success. It also means that I have continually been thwarted in my efforts to get the major government research organizations—the National Institutes of Health and the National Cancer Institute—involved in shark-cartilage research. The people I contacted said if it couldn't be done in a drug form, they weren't interested; they didn't work with natural products. The scientists whom I contacted would not speak on my behalf. With the peer system that exists, scientists are afraid of taking one false step because their peers may criticize them. On the other hand, I was raised to believe that unless you stick your neck out, you don't go forward. In light of the overwhelming evidence that shark cartilage has antiangiogenic properties and may have an effect on various diseases, how can I sit by idly?

When Eli Glatstein, M.D., chief of radiation oncology at Southwest Medical School, was asked by people affiliated with *60 Minutes* to look at before and after x-rays from the Cuban study, he said there were some cases in which the tumors got smaller, but added he'd like to see them get even smaller. He called for shark cartilage researchers to purify the material and find out what's responsible for the tumor regressions.

Many scientists, among them Carl Luer, point to a need to identify the active components in shark cartilage in order to understand their biological effects before we begin testing in humans. I believe, as I did from the moment CNN announced, "Shark cartilage cures cancer," that the important issues are:

- Is it nontoxic?
- Are there any side effects?
- Does it work?

It seems to me that if the answers to these questions are

affirmative, the next step is simple—use it—and learn more about how it works as you use it. With affirmative answers, scientific inquiry can take a back seat to the concerns of the suffering and dying patient and still get where it has to go.

Once toxicity testing proved negative—combined with the fact that the people of China have been eating shark-fin soup for years without side effects—I believed there was a moral imperative to begin testing in humans. As positive results from clinical trials mount, we now have a moral imperative to discover the active components and their underlying biological effects. This knowledge should expand treatment options in other arenas. In addition, it will hasten development of a synthetic drug, thereby safeguarding the shark population. It now appears that at least one government agency agrees: The FDA has granted an investigational new drug (IND) status to shark cartilage.

Currently, two companies have FDA approval to conduct pilot human clinical investigations. The studies will evaluate the safety and effectiveness of dry shark cartilage in reducing tumor size and improving related clinical characteristics in advanced prostate cancer and breast cancer. One company manufactures the product that was used in the Cuban trials. The second company has recently developed a product that appears to deliver even more of the active protein at less cost. In both cases, I made the initial contact with the FDA on behalf of the companies. (These are the first trials for which a natural product has been granted a full IND.) Another study of shark cartilage is being conducted by a physician in New Jersey under a treatment IND (see *Speeding the Drug Review Process* beginning on page 50). To find out if you are elegible to participate in one of these trials, have your physician contact NCI's PDQ, a computerized database. Patients may also call 800–4–CANCER themselves.

Before and during the trial period, manufacturers of shark cartilage products cannot make claims about the likelihood of the product's cancer-fighting potential or any other possible medical benefits. Until the trial results are available, shark cartilage will continue to be considered a dietary supplement.

THE CHANGING FACE OF SCIENCE

The story of my involvement with shark cartilage is really just one example of how the face of science has changed. The basic or pure scientist, once visualized as living in an ivory tower, has given way to the applied scientist, the researcher who more actively seeks practical application of his discoveries.

What is the reason for the change? Some of it is economic, stemming at least in part from the reduction of monies spent by the government on research. As one researcher has put it, the government cut the fat and is now "beginning to get the meat on the bones." Grant applications in the past twenty years have often received the label "approved but not funded." In these cases, no one is disputing the validity of the researcher or his protocol; no one is even questioning the need for the study; there simply isn't enough money to go around.

In a climate such as this, today's researchers often have to look elsewhere for funding. Some tailor their projects so they are attractive to industrial funding. Some turn to other governments (see *The Japanese Connection* beginning on page 76).

Some of the change in the scientific arena is due to public pressure. In the 1970s, people began to question whether the research path was too time-consuming and laden with scientific requirements. Some felt that NIH investigators did not have a sense of urgency and were primarily committed to the publication of papers. Then, too, the public felt scientists worked in an "ivory tower" because many investigators could not or would not take the time to translate scientific terminology into laymen's language. Not an endearing characteristic, and one that helped fuel the need for my first book.

The Japanese Connection

In American folklore, scientists are often depicted as bumbling, absent-minded professors covered in chalk dust or as wiry-haired madmen obsessed with accomplishing a goal. The truth is, of course, far less one-dimensional and far less extreme.

American scientists today come in many varieties; some are, no doubt, obsessive and many are absent-minded. These scientists and their colleagues work at universities, major corporations, and government agencies. Although the common denominator amongst them is supposed to be the quest for truth, it is more likely to be the quest for funds. Whether they seek grants from government or industry, or money from the chief operating officers of their companies, the one thing all scientists share is the need for money with which to conduct research. In our technological age, the cost of equipment—computers, laser Dopplers, electron microscopes—is practically prohibitive. And the cost of meeting government regulations doesn't help.

In the past several years, scientists at universities have been finding it particularly difficult to obtain funds. Government funding has been cut back and corporate support has not bridged the gap. In Japan, however, the picture has been different. The Japanese economy has been doing well, spurred on, in part, by discoveries made by American scientists. Consider, for instance, that the technology involved in the Trinitron television tube was developed by American engineers. The Japanese company SONY bought the patent and very successfully marketed their product. With this kind of success in hand, Japanese corporations have been quick to support research in America.

Japanese businesses and even the Japanese government have been funding research and making endowments at such places as Harvard (more than $94 million), Massachusetts Institute of Technology ($24.5 million), and the University of Michigan ($3 million). Other countries have also been eager to *get in on scientific research. In one recent year, MIT received approximately $13 million from foreign corporations; more than half of this money came from Japan.*

One of the researchers who has been involved in the "Japanese connection" is Judah Folkman, M.D., professor of surgery at Harvard Medical School and Children's Hospital. Dr. Folkman and his colleague, Donald Ingber, M.D., Ph.D., associate professor of pathology, had discovered a particular fungus's potential as an antiangiogenic agent while working under support from the National Institutes of Health. As has long been the practice among American scientists, the men hoped to isolate the agent in order to turn it into a drug. According to **The Boston Globe** *of January 3, 1994, Dr. Folkman said the process costs so much money that an industrial partner is necessary. The article reports that Dr. Folkman had unsuccessfully tried to interest United States pharmaceutical companies in angiogenesis research in 1986. At that time, a twelve-year $25 million contract with Monsanto Chemical Company that involved similar research had just expired. Takeda, a Japanese firm, offered its support and agreed to make the ensuing drug available in the United Sates first.*

According to the **Globe** *article, the fungus-derived drug is in early clinical trials under the auspices of the FDA. It is being tested against Kaposi's sarcoma and a variety of other cancers. In that article, Dr. Folkman is quoted as saying that the only alternative to taking a financial risk and developing a drug "is to make the discovery, publish it in* **Science** *or* **Nature***, then just hope somebody will do something about it." He pointed out, however, that "patients with cancer call frequently, and there is a certain pressure not to wait years and years."*

Waiting is probably easier for those scientists who, like their counterparts in folklore, stay in their ivory towers. They pursue their chosen paths while insulated from both the cries of the masses and the need to scratch for a buck.

IN CONCLUSION

Much has changed in science research, but much has stayed the same since the days of Pasteur and Lister. Those who have visions that separate them from the establishment must fight an uphill battle—a battle I've been proud to fight. And I have not stood alone. There are some researchers who believe that shark cartilage may be an effective cancer treatment, but it has primarily been those involved in alternative health care and the cancer victims themselves who have been behind shark cartilage.

Of course, the FDA's granting of the IND status for shark cartilage has been, so far, the highlight of my quest. It is a significant sign that the tree is starting to bend. And now that shark cartilage has moved into Phase II of the clinical trials, the jury will soon have a verdict. That verdict will leave someone with egg on his face. It may be me; it may be those scientists who have scorned me. Time will tell.

What is of the utmost importance is that the evidence be examined, the claims be tested, and the truth be known. That's all I have ever asked. Whatever the results of the current clinical trials, scientists, government agencies, and private individuals should work together to fight the real enemy—cancer. If we spend our time feuding, casting stones, and seeking personal gain, this important work cannot move forward, and people will continue to die.

6.

The Medical Establishment and Shark Cartilage

The goal of medicine as a social institution is to further, or to accomplish, the healing of society members who are sick, as well as prevent their getting sick in the first place. Central to an examination of the practical content of any system of medicine then should be its effectiveness in reducing the disease burden with the treated population over time.

—J. Warren Salmon, Ph.D.
Alternative Medicines

Over time, the "disease burden" of the population being treated for cancer has not been significantly reduced. In fact, the trauma and injuries resulting from conventional drugs and treatment are a major cause for the public's disillusionment with medical advances and one of the reasons for the growing interest in alternative medicine.

As the co-author of *Sharks Don't Get Cancer* and the spokes-man for shark cartilage therapy, I receive hundreds of calls and letters each month. People constantly ask how shark cartilage works, whether it can help them, and whether it has been approved by the FDA. I am not a medical doctor nor is anyone in my office, and we always tell people that up front. But it rarely stops the avalanche of questions as desperate people look for a solution, usually after all conventional therapies have failed and death is imminent.

I try to have others in my office steer these people to knowl-edgeable medical doctors. Out of compassion, I may talk with some people, again cautioning them that I am a researcher and the clearinghouse for information on shark cartilage, not a medical doctor. Frequently, as I discuss the anecdotal evidence from around the world—especially from the Cuban trials—and explain the probable mechanism behind shark cartilage's action, hope builds in the listener. I can hear it in the person's tone and words. Unfortunately, these people often find their hopes dashed by well-meaning physicians who seem to have the attitude, "Hurry up and do nothing." Oh, they may recommend surgery or radia-tion or chemotherapy, but research shows whether you do noth-ing at all or treat cancer with those modalities, the results will often be the same. So instead of considering the possibility that an alternative method may be a viable option, these doctors have patients do what amounts to nothing.

I have so often encountered "conventional" or traditional physicians whose attitude condemns a cancer patient that I almost want to cry when I hear the patient say the words, "Let me speak to my doctor." It is especially frustrating because I know that anything I say at that point will be misinterpreted. I always, in desperation, ask that the doctor phone me. I often even give out my private telephone number for such calls, but the doctors rarely call. In most cases, the next I hear, if I hear at all, is that the patient died. Whenever this happens, I remember a television interview I gave in Australia in April 1994.

I was interviewed by Allen Jones, whom I found to be a very bright interviewer. Late into the show, after we had discussed at length the concept behind the use of shark cartilage and the results we were getting, Allen referred to the issue of education. His statement has made a lasting impression on me: "Education is designed to open one's mind. Why is it that doctors and scientists who are so well-educated are so close-minded?" Maybe it's fear.

Perhaps doctors are afraid of lawsuits that might arise out of the use of nonconventional therapies. A doctor knows the chances of helping an advanced cancer patient with chemotherapy are minimal, but he also knows that if the patient dies, he will not be sued. He, however, fears that if he suggests a nonconventional therapy such as shark cartilage and the patient dies, three lawyers will be in his office the next day. Thus, *to protect themselves*, many doctors will not suggest shark cartilage therapy.

According to one health-care writer, those who reject alternative medicine out of hand are "unwilling to accept any belief that deviates from their own rigid party line." Therefore, good physicians might take a cue from good congresspeople; both, after all, are supposed to represent the public's best interests. Physicians and congressmen alike need to practice bipartisan politics, combining the best points from democratic and republican platforms or from traditional and alternative medicine. To best represent the needs of a people whose interests in alternative medicine are so obviously growing, physicians need to open their minds, become educated about alternative therapies, and discuss them with their patients. As the *Medical World News* put it in September 1993, "Physicians who care about their patients' well-being should support the treatment that is effective and causes no harm."

Fortunately, as the word gets around, some physicians are now telling patients that they have heard good things about shark cartilage, that it probably won't hurt, and that they would be pleased to monitor results for the patient.

GETTING THE WORD TO THE TRENCHES

I really believe that the physicians who are helping patients to battle cancer day in and day out should learn about alternatives such as shark cartilage. It's time for them to realize that there are other avenues than those explained by the pharmaceutical company's detail man. There are treatment modalities other than the strictly chemical drugs learned in medical schools.

James Forsythe, M.D., an oncologist and assistant clinical professor of internal medicine at the University of Nevada-Reno, says he has become more open-minded about alternative medicine because he's seen so many patients do better with it than they were expected to.

Consider, too, the words of Dr. Samuel Epstein, professor of occupational and environmental medicine at the University of Illinois School of Public Health in Chicago. In an article published in the October 1994 issue of *Working Woman*, he says, "The war on cancer has been dominated by powerful, interlocking professional and financial interests—with the highly profitable drug-development system at its hub—and that helps explain why treatment is still the priority, despite the fact that the ability to cure most cancers has not materially improved."

There are a handful of cancers that conventional treatments can reverse or manage very well, but the vast majority of cancers cannot be controlled with the accepted treatments. People using alternatives may fare better, or at least, no worse. In a study conducted with 117 terminal cancer patients at an American clinic, half the patients received conventional therapy and half received an alternative. It was found that the length of survival did not differ between the two groups. The researchers involved recommended, therefore, that future studies compare patients receiving treatment with patients receiving only pain relievers. When studies such as this were conducted in Europe, it was found that *people who do nothing have the same life expectancy* as those receiving treatment.

Such studies might put an end to what author Stephen Barret calls "the war over cancer therapies" in which "both sides often describe the opposition as a malevolent monolith. Thus, the cancer establishment has characterized the alternative and adjunctive cancer therapies as the work of quacks preying on desperate and credulous cancer victims, while the proponents of alternative therapies have depicted established therapies as the cut, burn, and poison therapies of a cynical and profit-driven conspiracy."

TIME AND TIDE TURN SOME AROUND

It's not surprising that when I first started speaking to the public, there were almost no M.D.s in the audience. Now, a fair number of talks are given to medical organizations. And when TV's Dr. Bob Arnot became *Good Housekeeping's* "Family Doctor," he mentioned shark cartilage in his first column. He noted how popular an alternative treatment it was in 1993. He went on to explain that researchers had identified a component of shark cartilage that might prevent the spread of cancers by cutting off their blood supply.

Dr. Arnot is just one example of the many physicians who have, in fact, been receptive to shark cartilage. Perhaps it is those who are in the trenches with the victims of cancer who are likely to seek a "better way." Doctors desperate for an effective alternative to the current methods of fighting the disease are willing to listen. I have, therefore, been invited to speak about my research by the oncology staffs at several leading hospitals including the University of California-Irvine and the Montefiore and Albert Einstein Medical School in the Bronx, New York.

My first talk before a major medical organization was presented at New York City's Metropolitan Hospital Center, a teaching affiliate of New York Medical College, in May 1993. On that occasion, the Cuban physicians who had run the clinical

Advice Has Its Advantages

One of the delights of traveling is eating—sampling regional foods, experiencing local delicacies. So Wallace "Wally" Bothum and his wife, Davella "Mickey," of Gresham, Oregon, weren't surprised at the weight they gained during a year's travels around the United States.

At the end of their trip in November of 1993, Wally and Mickey returned to their winter home in Hawaii. They soon found that working in the yard and swimming daily helped them lose most of the weight they had gained over the previous year; but Mickey's tummy kept getting bigger. During the months that followed, Mickey realized that she wasn't able to eat much before feeling full. In April, she made an appointment to see the doctor.

An ultrasound, a CAT scan, and a CA-125 test confirmed the couple's worst fears. Mickey had cancer. (A CA-125 is a blood test that can detect the presence of ovarian cancer. A normal reading on the test ranges from 0 to 35; Mickey's reading was more than 3,000.) The primary cancer site was determined to be the ovary, but the cancer had spread extensively in the abdominal area and was considered inoperable. The doctors in Hawaii predicted that Mickey had three to six months to live.

"When one has a terminal disease," says Wally, "advice comes from everywhere: 'Try this and that.' We were well aware of the charlatans and passed shark cartilage off as one of those desperate cure-alls. That is, until we heard first-hand about the experience of Bruce Allen, whom I've known personally for over fifty years." Bruce had recently been diagnosed with prostate cancer that had metastasized to the bone. Members of the medical profession didn't give him much chance to live. Dying and in much pain, Bruce started taking shark cartilage. Today his pain is gone and the cancer is in remission. (See A Battle Is Won, But the War Goes On beginning on page 109.)

Having known, respected, and trusted Bruce for so long, Mickey and Wally felt they had to take a chance on shark cartilage.

They returned to their home in Oregon and Mickey began taking the cartilage immediately while under the care of oncologist Ivan P. Uhle, M.D. The couple did not tell the oncologist that Mickey was using the cartilage.

Mickey had two chemotherapy treatments at three-week intervals and was taking shark cartilage orally on a daily basis. During that time, she lost twelve inches from her middle.

Dr. Uhle soon felt it was time to remove Mickey's ovaries; he ordered one more session of chemotherapy, following which surgery was performed on July 19, 1994. Although the oncologist believed that Mickey was cancer-free after the surgery, the pathologist's report would be the final word.

During the biopsy, the pathologist discovered some white cells that baffled him. He sent the slides to a doctor who was studying ovarian cancer at the medical school. When the Bothums heard about this, they decided to tell the doctors that Mickey had been taking shark cartilage.

According to Wally, Dr. Uhle responded to the news by saying, "Shark cartilage? That's interesting! I have a memo on my desk from the National Health Institute wanting information I may have about patients who have been using shark cartilage." Wally reports that Dr. Uhle went on to say, "Well, we know one thing for sure, Mickey had a very serious disease and she doesn't have it any more. Whatever you did, keep on doing it!" Dr. Uhle also took Bruce Allen's phone number and contacted him to learn more about his experience with shark cartilage.

Dr. Uhle had planned for Mickey to have two more treatments with chemotherapy following the surgery. After one treatment, she told him she wouldn't take any more. Dr. Uhle ordered another CAT scan and another CA-125 ovarian cancer test, which confirmed that Mickey was in remission. The CA-125 reading was now 7! When Wally asked the oncologist if he thought Mickey's remission had been rapid, Dr. Uhle said, "Yes, because she had only three treatments. If patients respond at all, it usually takes six to nine treatments, and sometimes up to a year."

Dr. Uhle told Mickey, "You don't have any more cancer, you're clean," and agreed that she need have no more chemotherapy. The pathology report showed the cancer cells were dead— those white cells that had baffled the pathologist turned out to be dead cancer cells—and a subsequent CA-125 reading was 3. According to Wally, more chemotherapy at this point would have been like "beating a dead horse."

In November 1994, Mickey had been pronounced "cured." "We don't know for certain why or what caused Mickey's rapid remission," says Wally. "But between God, the expertise of Dr. Uhle, and shark cartilage, a cure resulted. We are grateful and thankful for all, whatever part they played."

---

trial featured on *60 Minutes* presented their findings to an audience of approximately fifty physicians. The proceedings were chaired by Steven Holt, M.D., who told the assembled doctors and some members of the press, "Claims for shark cartilage generate zeal on the one hand and skepticism on the other. I think what we have to do is look very critically at all of the observations given any new therapeutic option."

Dr. Holt's words have been echoed by Barrie R. Cassileth, Ph.D., adjunct professor of medicine at the University of North Carolina and consulting professor of community and family medicine at Duke University. In the August 1994 issue of *Oncology Times*, Dr. Cassileth is quoted as saying, "The challenge to oncologists is keeping patients' goals realistic and keeping the door open to discussion."

One doctor who has had an open-door policy is Joshua Atiba, M.D., an oncologist at the University of California-Irvine. He is convinced that shark cartilage works. On February 11, 1994, the *Seattle Post-Intelligencer* quoted Dr. Atiba as saying, "It's not hocus pocus. It inhibits the growth of blood vessels in tumors."

But other physicians have expressed skepticism if not outright hostility. Dr. Basel Yanes, an oncologist and medical director of the David L. Rike Cancer Center at Miami Valley Hospital in Ohio is "wary" of shark cartilage therapy because the claims seem "too good to be true." He feels that there is no scientific evidence that shark cartilage is an effective cancer treatment. Dr. James F. Holland, an oncologist at Mt. Sinai Medical Center in New York, was interviewed by Dr. Jay Adlersberg on WABC-TV's Eyewitness News in April 1995. Dr. Holland said, "Until shark cartilage is shown to be inactive, which I expect it will be—and it will have to be looked at by people other than the proponents who have a very substantial financial motivation to have it be active—I don't think anybody should take shark cartilage." What a sweeping generalization! Dr. Holland doesn't want *anybody* to take a completely safe, nontoxic food product. Why? Because it *may* not be active. Dr. Adlersberg went on to say that Dr. Holland's fears are based on the feeling that "people who use unproven cures deny themselves the chance to get better with more proven means."

The medical establishment's negative feelings have actually delayed our learning all of the facts about shark cartilage as a therapy. Because few physicians have been willing to work with patients, statistics about shark cartilage's medicinal value are slow in coming. These physicians may fear being ostracized by their peers—perhaps even losing their jobs—if they become involved with an alternative therapy. In fact, the second set of Phase II clinical trials approved by the FDA have been delayed because of difficulty in finding a hospital in which the trials can be run. Although a physician at Shriner's Hospital in Chicago had been eager to oversee the trials, he bowed out when establishment pressure was brought to bear. I then had to find a physician who could—and would—oversee trials at a different hospital. Thankfully, José Gonzalez, M.D., a prominent urology oncologist at William Beaumont Hospital in Detroit, Michigan, has agreed to head the trials with the help of Ananias Diokno, M.D., chief of urology.

Dr. Gonzalez took the time to thoroughly research shark cartilage and then decided that studies of its efficacy were important. Unfortunately, it appears that many doctors are ignorant about research into shark cartilage and, possibly, about the limited success conventional therapies have had in the treatment of most cancers. For instance, many physicians don't realize that with the FDA's granting of two INDs, shark cartilage moved from an "unproven cure" to an experimental one. Secondly, in my first book and in all of my speaking appearances, I continually entreat patients to continue with their conventional treatments.

When I spoke to the Breast Cancer Action Group in Burlington, Vermont, the *Burlington Free Press* carried an article that told the story of a forty-five-year-old woman who had been diagnosed with breast cancer and had been taking shark cartilage for two years. The woman said it had kept a tumor in her lung from growing, but added, "My doctor won't admit that cartilage is the reason the tumor stopped growing. He said the claims that are made about shark cartilage don't make sense." But physicians are not the only ones who have expressed skepticism.

William Jarvis, president of the National Center Against Health Fraud, agrees. He says there's no reason to believe that shark cartilage works because sharks do get tumors, even in their cartilage. Dr. Adlersberg chose to end his broadcast with the words, "By the way, Dr. Holland says sharks do get cancer." The sharks-*do*-get-cancer issue was also jumped on by people at *Scientific American*, which ran an article in September 1993 headed "Sharks Do Get Cancer" (see reprint of article beginning on page 23). I have always recognized that, yes, sharks do get cancer, but on the order of one in a million, a number too miniscule to pick fights over.

Even physicians usually considered friendly to alternative medicine have sometimes attacked my work. A good example is Alan Gaby, M.D., an editor for *The Townsend Letter*, an important alternative medicine periodical. To my knowledge, he had never spoken with me nor had he attended my recent presentations. He had heard me speak a number of years earlier, before the human evidence developed. Based on that, he wrote several very negative articles about my work. Recently, at my request, he has finally spoken to me and to Neal Adelman, M.D., who has treated a large number of cancer patients with shark cartilage and other therapies. Since then, the incidence of negative articles about shark cartilage written by Dr. Gaby has stopped.

OPEN MINDS SHAKE BUREAUCRACY

The open-minded attitude of some people involved in health care has caused tensions within the Office of Alternative Medicine (OAM). It has been said that one of the reasons Joseph Jacobs, M.D., the first director of OAM, resigned in September 1994 was because of the controversy over shark cartilage (see detailed account, beginning on page 55).

In September 1993, an ad hoc advisory panel recommended that OAM start—"without delay"—to investigate three forms of therapy, among them "the use of shark cartilage infusions in patients with cancer." Leanna Standish, Ph.D., research director at Bastyr College of Natural Health Sciences in Seattle, Washington, was among the most moving of the panel members. As related in the *Journal of the American Medical Association* in September 1993, Dr. Standish said that each and every day she is asked by women with breast cancer about the efficacy of taking shark cartilage; she told OAM she wanted to know the answers. Gar Hildenbrand, executive director of the Gerson Institute in Bonita, California, seconded her plea, imploring the OAM to get the information people need.

Fortunately, there is some good news. Under its current director, Dr. Wayne B. Jonas, the OAM has become more focused in its research on alternative treatments. Such positive steps should elicit answers.

IN CONCLUSION

Establishment of the Office of Alternative Medicine was a positive step in recognizing that alternative therapies may hold the key to the effective treatment of various diseases that aren't being controlled by conventional methods. Perhaps these methods keep cancer patients so busy with treatment that they don't have enough time to ask the right questions: Are these therapies really extending their lives, or are they putting patients through needless hell?

Should we not take a step back and take an objective look at the state of conventional cancer treatments? Should we not say that it might be wiser to keep our options open? If it is possible that shark cartilage holds an answer, should we not at least say, "Let's give it a chance"?

7.

Cancer Studies

Cancer [L. a crab, a cancer. CANC-] A general term frequently used to indicate any of various types of malignant neoplasms, most of which invade surrounding tissues, may metastasize to several sites, and are likely to recur after attempted removal and to cause death of the patient unless adequately treated; any carcinoma or sarcoma (or other malignant neoplasm), but, in ordinary usage, especially the former.

—Stedman's Medical Dictionary

Cancer . . . malignant . . . metastasize. These are words that make us shudder in fear. They are words that mean the "death of the patient unless adequately treated." Yet "adequate" treatment is usually as frightening as the disease itself. Chemotherapy, radiation, surgery—there is little comfort to be found in these words. It is not, then, surprising that researchers have long sought another way—a better way.

ANTIANGIOGENESIS—A THEORY OFFERS HOPE

One of the most promising theories of recent times may well be Dr. Judah Folkman's hypothesis regarding antiangiogenesis.

Since tumors cannot grow without a blood network to nourish them and to remove waste products, stopping the development of blood vessels may be a potential cancer therapy.

A very exciting feature of antiangiogenic agents is that they are theoretically less likely to precipitate drug resistance than the cytotoxic drugs now used in chemotherapy. The vascular endothelial cells from which capillaries sprout do not seem to have the multi-drug resistant gene except perhaps for those endothelial cells in the brain and testes. Again, this is one of Dr. Folkman's hypotheses.

TURNING HOPE INTO REALITY

Using shark cartilage as an antiangiogenic agent became my dream after I met John Prudden, M.D., Med.Sc.D, a Harvard-trained surgeon who was an early pioneer in the medical uses of cartilage. Today's surgical texts routinely include information on the preparation of cartilage for use as an accelerator of wound-healing, a treatment that Dr. Prudden experimented with in 1960. Dr. Prudden was also the first person ever to conduct research in which cancer patients were successfully treated using cartilage as an immune-system stimulator and mild angiogenesis inhibitor (see page 10).

After learning of Dr. Prudden's study and of the work Drs. Langer and Lee had conducted at MIT (see discussion beginning on page 9), I decided to see if whole shark cartilage was biologically active. I spent many years creating a product that would be as pure as possible. Finding a way to dry and then pulverize shark cartilage without rendering the protein fibers ineffective was a major problem. At least one of the proteins that is active as an angiogenesis inhibitor is denatured (rendered inactive) if processing temperatures are elevated. The proteins are also inactivated if they are treated with solvents like acetone or submitted to strong acids for extended periods.

Particle size is another consideration. Shark cartilage particles must be absorbed into the system as quickly as possible to prevent the protein from being digested by proteolytic enzymes, which would break down the protein into ineffective constituent amino acids or small polypeptides. The angiogenesis-inhibiting properties of shark cartilage are in the preformed or native protein found in the stringlike fibers in the cartilage. I spent many years, much effort, and a great deal of money getting the cartilage ready for use.

Once I felt my goal had been achieved, I decided to find physicians who would be willing to test shark cartilage on patients. I was informed by several distinguished physicians and scientists that there was no point in trying to interest American researchers who investigate only those drugs that can be patented.

While scores of people die and scores more suffer from the effects of traditional cancer therapies, scientists continue to believe that identification, purification, and synthesis of the protein(s) responsible for angiogenesis is the *only* way to go. Nothing could be further from the truth.

These three scientific pathways (identification, purification, and synthesis) might actually prove to be blind alleys in the attempt to produce an antiangiogenic drug. First, there is the problem of isolating the protein or proteins without destroying them. Proteins are easily denatured by various chemicals and various manufacturing processes, especially pulverization and sterilization, which can generate a lot of heat. The problem can perhaps be best explained by using the common egg. The white of an egg, the albumin protein, is soluble in water until it is heated. Heat causes the white to coagulate. When it coagulates, it changes from colorless to white, from liquid to solid, from water soluble to water insoluble. The white still has the same amount of protein, but its form and possible activity have been materially changed. Its chemical analysis is the same, but its biological activity and appearance are completely different.

In addition to changing the protein, isolation removes it from its environment. In the case of shark cartilage, isolating the angiogenesis-inhibiting protein would mean separating it from the mucopolysaccharide that has the anti-inflammatory effect. Would the resulting substance be as effective? And can any of the several proteins responsible for inhibition of angiogenesis be separated from the others without changing its efficacy? (We believe that there are at least four proteins responsible for the full antiangiogenesis effect.) How long will it take to find out? Another ten months or ten years? How many people will develop degenerative diseases while the investigation continues? How many will die while a nonchemical, natural, whole product might be saving lives? Remember, Drs. Langer and Folkman convinced themselves that giving cartilage orally would not work because the acidic stomach would denature the angiogenesis-inhibiting protein or break it down into small noneffective peptides. They never even tested it. Recent research into digestion indicates that their belief may have been erroneous (see pages 158–163).

Furthermore, isolation of antiangiogenic proteins has proven to be difficult. The properties of the original protein extracts were inconsistent and much of the 1970s was spent trying to develop assays. A breakthrough did not come until the late 1980s. Now, at least ten angiogenic factors have been purified, but we still have no angiogenesis-fighting drugs. Several of these factors exhibit some toxicity, which would be quite dangerous if the drug were taken over a prolonged period of time.

EARLY CLINICAL TRIALS

Because of the American research establishment's mindset against "natural" medicines, I went to other countries in pursuit of trials to test shark cartilage. The first breakthrough came in

1985 at the prestigious Jules Bordet Cancer Institute in Brussels when studies conducted with mice showed that shark cartilage was nontoxic and effective when orally administered.

The first human clinical trials were conducted in Mexico where seven out of eight terminal cancer patients had positive responses to the therapy. In these seven cases, tumor sizes diminished 40 to 100 percent in seventy days or less. After eleven weeks, one person had withdrawn from the program, three had attained a 60 percent reduction in tumor size, and three were tumor-free. Small-scale trials were then conducted in Panama where the results were equally impressive. The results of these studies gave me the fuel needed to generate the first large-scale human study in Cuba.

In the Cuban trial, twenty-nine terminal patients (those with six months or less to live) who had not received any therapy for five or six weeks prior to the trial, used shark cartilage as their only treatment. Initially, each patient received 60 grams per day of shark cartilage via retention enemas. After six weeks, the same dose was given orally or rectally; this dose was maintained for the duration of the sixteen-week study. Following the study, patients took a maintenance dose of 20 grams daily.

When the initial phase of the study concluded in January 1993, twenty patients had been participating for the entire sixteen weeks. Almost 40 percent of them experienced significant improvement in their conditions. The remaining 60 percent included one woman who withdrew from the study and two who had died of conditions that were not related to their cancers. Another woman had colon cancer that had metastasized to the liver; at the end of sixteen weeks, her liver condition appeared to have worsened. Two patients with metastatic breast cancer had reported feeling less pain during the study but died just before the sixteen-week evaluation was completed. In three other cases, there was initial shrinkage of the tumors, which subsequently showed regrowth.

Many of the patients had significant improvement in their

conditions. Furthermore, the consensus among the participating physicians was that even in the cases where tumor shrinkage was negligible, the quality of life improved. Patients exhibited an increase of body weight, appetite, and mobility. Their lung capacity improved, their psychological base improved. In addition, there was significant amelioration of pain, which is experienced by virtually all terminal cancer patients, of whom 50 to 90 percent require narcotic medication.

One way in which the patients in the Cuban trial were evaluated was with the Karnofsky Performance Scale (see Table 7.1). This scale, which numerically rates the patient's ability for normal activity or the need for care, confirmed that the subjects were able to do more things and do them more easily than before the treatment. For instance, one man in the study who had been at death's door with prostate cancer was able to run daily following treatment.

José Menendez, M.D., Ph.D., senior professor of internal medicine at Havana University, consulting professor of internal medicine at the National Autonomous University of Managua, Nicaragua, member of the advisory group of the Cuban Minister of Health, deputy dean for medical practice and research at Havana's Higher Institute of Military Medicine, led the team of five Cuban doctors. José Fernandez-Britto, M.D., Ph.D., senior professor of pathology with the World Health Organization (WHO), chief of the Pathologic Anatomy Department at Dr. Carlos J. Finlay Military University Hospital, consulting professor of the Rudolf Vicchow Pathology Institute at Humbold University in Germany, and vice president of the Pan-American Pathological Association, was in charge of pathology.

During the trial, nine of the original twenty-nine patients died during the first seventeen weeks. Although they had been improving, as evidenced by pathological slides, their diseases were so far advanced that even though they were winning the battle, they lost the war. Six more have since died, but not of cancer; they died of heart attacks, accidents, pneumonia—

Table 7.1 The Karnofsky Performance Scale

The Karnofsky Performance Scale numerically rates the patient's ability for normal activity or the need for care. The description of each ten-point increment in the 0–100 point scale is presented below.

Rating	Ability
100	Normal physical and mental capabilities; no complaints; no evidence of disease.
90	Able to carry on normal activity; minor signs and symptoms of disease.
80	Normal activity with effort; some signs and symptoms of disease.
70	Cares for self; unable to carry on normal activity or do active work.
60	Requires occasional assistance but is able to care for most personal needs.
50	Requires considerable assistance and frequent medical care.
40	Disabled; requires special care and assistance.
30	Severely disabled; hospitalization is indicated, although death is not imminent.
20	Very sick; hospitalization is necessary; active supportive treatment is necessary.
10	Moribund; fatal processes progressing rapidly.
0	Death.

things other than cancer. Today, three and a half years after the start of the study, fourteen of the subjects are alive and well— riding bicycles, running, and walking—enjoying the normal quality of life so often denied with conventional cancer therapies. These patients who had been given up for dead are alive and functioning as normal people, and their only therapy was shark cartilage (see photos on pages 100–101).

The Cuban study was especially significant because the

patients were hospitalized throughout the trial. They were given the medication, and we know they took it and took nothing else. In most clinical trials, patients are sent home with an active medication or a placebo, told what to do, and when to report back. The number of these patients who actually take the pills or who simply flush them down the toilet and tell the doctors otherwise is an unknown factor. Recently, two women who had been subjects in the Tamoxafen trials admitted to having shared each other's pills to ensure that neither of them took the placebo only. Problems such as these were eliminated from the Cuban trials.

Hospitalization of subjects also meant that we were able to obtain some blood studies and x-rays. At six weeks, both the blood studies and films showed improvement. The physicians noted that there were more immune bodies in the circulation, causing a stronger immunological response than is typically seen in cancer patients. Normally, advanced cancer patients exhibit an unresponsive immunological pattern. This means they lack the ability to ward off diseases caused by organisms or anything else that the immune system normally recognizes as a foreign body. These important immunological markers seem directly related to the administration of shark cartilage.

One of the most striking cases in the Cuban trial was of Frankie, the woman whose thirty-five-pound ovarian tumor was considered inoperable because of its large size and because it had grown into the bone of her pelvis. After twenty-three weeks of shark cartilage therapy, she was approved for surgery. The operation revealed that the tumor had detached from the pelvis and had shrunk by 23 percent. At the time of removal, the tumor weighed twenty-four pounds and was completely encapsulated and necrotic (comprised of dead tissue). Interestingly, the surgery was practically bloodless. Photos of Frankie taken before and after her surgery are displayed on page 101.

Following the Cuban study, Drs. Menendez and Fernandez-Britto came to America to meet with the press and with interested members of the medical profession. The physicians had not expected to obtain visas because of the strained relationship between Cuba and the United States and because Dr. Menendez is a senior military officer. However, with the help of Senator Bill Bradley's office staff, the visas were obtained.

The first conference was held at Metropolitan Hospital Center on the upper east side of Manhattan early in May 1993. Organized by the Hospital's chief of the department of dermatology, Philip Don, M.D., the conference was moderated by Stephen Holt, M.D., then chief of gastroenterology at Long Island College Hospital. At the conference, some participants expressed the feeling that shark cartilage is a major breakthrough in effective cancer treatment" and may result in a prescribable treatment in the United States within two to three years. Hopefully, both a prescription form of shark cartilage and a health-food supplement will be available to the public in the future.

Much of the excitement was generated by the fact that the studies to date have been conducted only on patients who have not responded to conventional treatment. Although conventional medicine offered them no recourse, they experienced significant improvement with shark cartilage therapy. The improvement in the Cuban patients was so dramatic that Dr. Menendez refers to the trial as "the happiest experience of my medical career."

The availability of information from a pathologist was in itself a significant aspect of the Cuban study. Autopsies were performed on victims of breast, bladder, and prostate cancer, and on tissue from lymph node metastasis, primary metastasis, and liver metastasis. Dr. Fernandez-Britto compared the tissues of those who had used shark cartilage with tissues of those who had died of the same disease and had not used shark cartilage. Some interesting observations were noted.

For instance, fibrinogen—a precursor for the fibrous protein that is involved in blood clotting—was present in the tissue

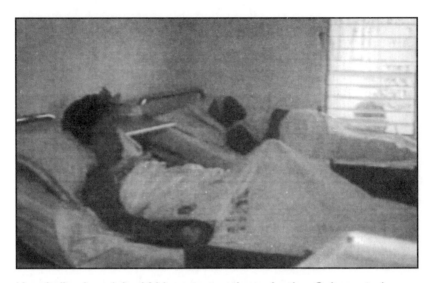

Hospitalized and bedridden, two patients in the Cuban study are shown here at the onset of the trial. All of the participants were considered terminal with less than six months to live.

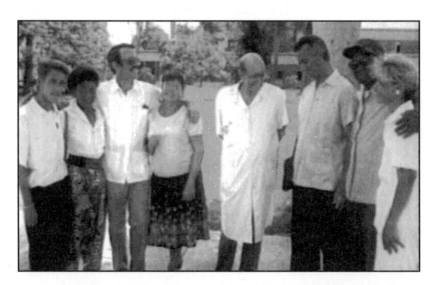

Two years after the study, some of the participants are pictured here with oncologist Dr. José Menendez (third from left) and pathologist Dr. José Fernandez-Britto (fifth from the left). To date, all of those who completed the study are alive and well.

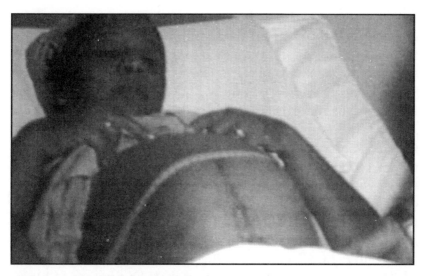

Frankie, as she appeared at the beginning of the study with a thirty-five pound ovarian tumor. After twenty-three weeks of shark cartilage therapy, the tumor had shrunk to twenty-four pounds and was removed.

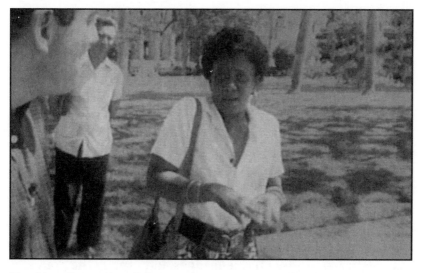

Frankie, alive and well, is seen here two years after the study.

samples of those who had been taking the shark cartilage. Not normally found in cancer tissue, fibrinogen is seen beginning to invade, encapsulate, and replace the cancer cells in the slides shown in Figures 7.1 and 7.2. The patients from whom these tissue samples were taken died; however, the presence of the fibrous tissue indicates the shark cartilage had been working.

In addition to the autopsy samples, a number of biopsies (examination of living tissue) were also performed during the course of the Cuban trial. Figures 7.3 and 7.4 show before and after tissue samples from one patient in the study with prostate cancer. Figure 7.3 shows the cancer cells, which have taken over the tissue, before the patient began the shark cartilage treatment. These truly formed cancer cells became weak and diffuse, as seen in Figure 7.4, after the therapy had begun.

Dr. Fernandez-Britto also noted that the number of blood vessels in connective tissue increases at the same time the blood vessels in the tumor mass decrease. The Cuban physicians and I refer to this phenomenon as "the theory of modulation."

THE THEORY OF MODULATION

Normally, tumors are particularly well vascularized at the periphery (outer edge). It is, in fact, the presence of these blood vessels that permits various anticancer therapies to approach the tumor. Necrosis or cell death commonly occurs at the center of the tumor because the blood supply does not reach the core. In fact, the innermost part of a tumor is so far from the closest blood vessel that the exchange of nutrients, oxygen, and carbon dioxide does not occur at the center. In autopsies of shark cartilage users, however, Dr. Fernandez-Britto observed necrosis of those tumor cells that are in contact with the connective tissue. This connective tissue bridges and repairs the area and does not usually have a blood supply.

Autopsies also revealed few blood vessels in the tumors but

double the amount in the fibrous tissue that developed as scar tissue. Vessel growth is directly proportional to the total fibrovascular growth. Dr. Fernandez-Britto found that in patients treated with shark cartilage, the tumors had been walled off and surrounded—encapsulated—by unusually large amounts of fibrous tissue that had its own blood supply as seen in Figure 7.2. It was determined that the connective tissue rapidly walls off the tumor and replaces that mass, often in less than fourteen weeks.

The pathologist hypothesizes that shark cartilage plays some role in modulating angiogenesis; it inhibits the growth of new blood vessels into the tumor mass while augmenting the blood vessels in the connective tissue that appears to encapsulate the tumor. He says, "Shark cartilage stimulates the development of blood vessels in the connective tissue surrounding the tumor cells, producing an angiogenic effect. As a result, an abundant dense fibrosis (fiberlike connective tissue that occurs in scar tissue) is observed, limiting the growth of the tumor cells and yielding peripheral necrosis, diminishing the size of the tumor."

In other words, we're seeing enhancement of angiogenesis in the healthy tissue and inhibition in the cancerous tissue. Says Dr. Fernandez-Britto, "I've never seen a reaction like this before." The evidence, obtained by microscopic examination of tissues, suggests that shark cartilage modulates angiogenesis rather than inhibits it.

The conference moderator, pointing to the measurable effect seen in the slides of autopsied tissue, commented that the clinical effects seen in the trial are "not explicable by chance." The reactions in the fibrous tissue where such changes are not commonly seen "has to be related to the administration of shark cartilage." Similar reactions were heard at meetings held at the University of Texas M.D. Anderson Cancer Center in Houston, Texas, and at the University of Chicago, the Princess Margaret Medical Center in Toronto, and at Southwest Texas University in San Marcos.

Area of
cancer cells
(black dots)

Fibrous tissue
(invading and
replacing
cancer cells)

Areas of
cancer cells

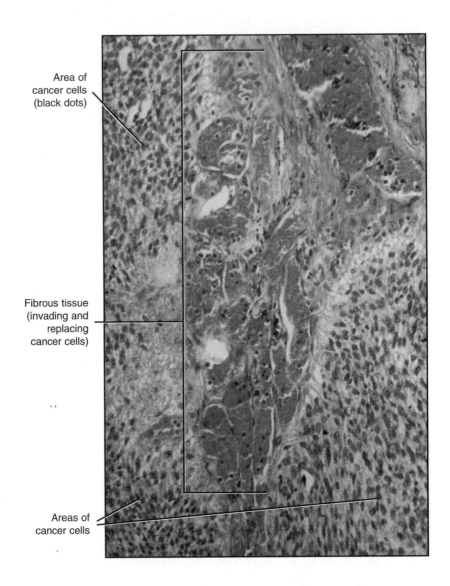

Figure 7.1.   Fibrous Tissue Invading Cancer Cells.
Slide of autopsied tissue shows cancer cells being invaded and replaced by
fibrous tissue. Tissue sample is from patient who had just begun shark
cartilage therapy.

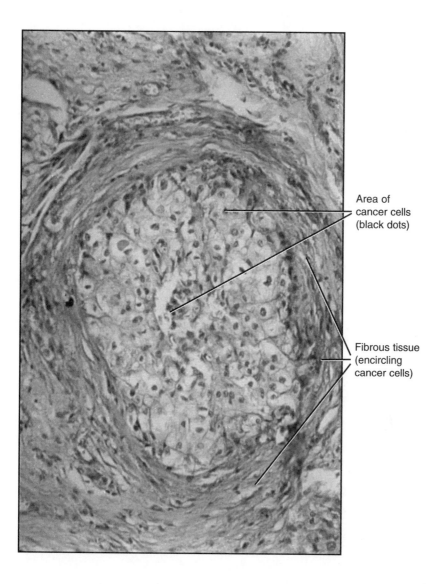

Area of
cancer cells
(black dots)

Fibrous tissue
(encircling
cancer cells)

Figure 7.2. Fibrous Tissue Encapsulating Cancer Cells.
Autopsied tissue shows cancer cells being encircled by fibrous tissue. Such encapsulation will eventually cut off the cancer cells' blood supply, resulting in their death. Tissue sample is from patient who had just started shark cartilage treatment.

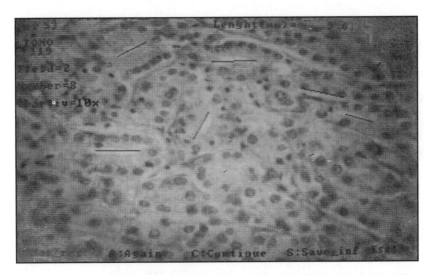

Figure 7.3.   Prostate-Cancer Tissue Before Shark Cartilage Therapy.
Biopsied tissue shows cancerous prostate tissue of patient at the onset of
the Cuban trial. Numerous cancer cells (black dots) are present.*

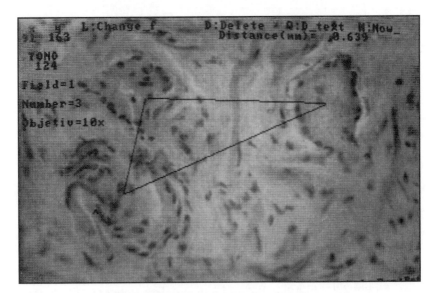

Figure 7.4.   Prostate-Cancer Tissue After Shark Cartilage Therapy.
Biopsied tissue from same patient as in Figure 7.3 after shark cartilage treatment
had begun. Note difference in the cancer cells, which are weak and diffuse.*

* *Note*: Pathologist's computer-generated markings are also present.

It is interesting to note that the concept of modulation is not without precedent. There is evidence from other researchers that different tissues can react in different ways to the same stimulator. For instance, research conducted in the department of surgery at Metropolitan Hospital Center by Norman Ackerman, M.D., Ph.D., and Roger Jacobs, Ph.D., revealed differing effects of epinephrine, a drug that constricts blood vessels. In experimental liver tumors, epinephrine was shown to increase blood flow within tumor tissues while decreasing blood flow in surrounding normal liver tissue.

Joseph Madri of the Yale University School of Medicine in Connecticut points to one growth factor's (TGF-beta) ability to significantly inhibit cell proliferation *in vitro* but induce angiogenesis *in vivo*. He says the materials outside the cell body itself, the extracellular matrix or materials that occupy the space between cells and bind them together to form a tissue, may influence a factor. The extracellular matrix in tumor tissue is different from that in healthy tissue.

More evidence of the modulation concept may be seen in the fact that the layer of cells lining blood vessels (endothelial cells) produce both plasminogen (an enzyme that converts the fibrin in blood clots to soluble products) activator and plasminogen inhibitor. Research also reveals that blood flow itself is variable: sometimes steady, sometimes pulsing; sometimes turbulent, sometimes nonturbulent. Each variation has a different effect on such things as cell shape, cell proliferation, and calcium levels of endothelial cells.

Consider the ideas of Rakesh Jain, Ph.D., professor of radiation oncology at Harvard Medical School, who believes blood vessels may provide information for treating cancer. In an article in the magazine *Biotechnology*, Dr. Jain reports that cancer therapies have been focused on cancer *cells* for thirty years. He believes it is time to consider blood vessels and interstitial space as therapeutic avenues.

CURRENT STATUS OF SHARK CARTILAGE TRIALS

Early in March 1994, the FDA granted final approval for Phase II human clinical trials on the effectiveness of shark cartilage as a cancer therapy (see page 72). The FDA was cooperative and approval came relatively quickly, due in part to the positive attitude of Dr. Gregory Burke, who is now retired from his post as head of the Division of Oncology and Pulmonary Drug Products.

Being conducted in New Jersey, these trials deal with advanced breast and prostate (stage IV) tumors. The FDA protocol requires that only those for whom at least two other treatments (i.e., radiation and chemotherapy, or two forms of chemotherapy) have failed be included in these shark cartilage trials. In addition, the presence of measurable metastatic tumors must be confirmed. Many other criteria, such as the names of the physicians involved, the hospital, and the members of the institutional review board, are carefully spelled out in the official IND. In the first stage of the trial, fourteen breast cancer and fourteen prostate cancer patients will complete a twenty-week study. Eventually, twenty patients will be enrolled in each group. Successful results with the first study may lead to a second and possibly a third larger study.

In April 1995, an IND was awarded to a second company for clinical trials. In this group of trials, fourteen patients with incurable prostate cancer and fourteen AIDS patients with Kaposi's sarcoma (a form of cancer in which irregular-shaped tumor cells cling to the linings of some blood vessels) will be the subjects. The two companies that received FDA approval represent two specific shark cartilage products, each of which is manufactured in its own specific way. It is important to note that the FDA has not approved testing of generic shark cartilage.

While Phase II clinical trials are being conducted at hospitals in Livingston, New Jersey, and in Detroit, Michigan, excitement about the therapeutic potential of shark cartilage is spanning the

A Battle Is Won, But the War Goes On

In 1983, the world turned upside down for Bruce Allen. That's when the sixty-six-year-old was diagnosed with prostatic cancer. After a radical prostectomy was performed, Bruce's life got back on target. He did quite well for ten years and then began to experience severe bone pain. Very high PSA (prostate specific antigen) levels were identified. (Serum PSA levels rise when a prostatic tumor is present.) CAT scans and bone scans revealed evidence of recurrent metastatic prostatic carcinoma in the bone. More than a dozen sites in Bruce's body were identified as "hot."

In July 1993, Bruce underwent a bilateral orchiectomy (removal of testes). But he wasn't leaving his life solely in the hands of surgeons. Three days before the scheduled surgery, he had started taking shark cartilage. For two days, he took 4.5 grams per day. By the day of his surgery, the excruciating pain in his bones was gone. But pain wasn't the only enemy Bruce was fighting. Laboratory reports had revealed metastases in his shoulders, sacrum, right hip, and left thigh. Patients with prostatic cancer that has metastasized usually live an average of two-and-a-half years. However, Bruce's bony metastases had been spreading rapidly and doctors did not expect him to live more than a few months.

After his surgery, Bruce added more ammunition in his battle for survival, gradually increasing his daily shark cartilage dose from 4.5 grams to 60 grams in January, then to 120 grams in March, and finally to 150–160 grams in August. Within three months of beginning shark cartilage therapy, bone scans confirmed bony metastasis control and reversal.

By October, Bruce's medical records indicated that three of the previously identified sites of metastasis were less hot while two others were a bit worse. No new areas of involvement were identified. In March, the doctor's notation read, "Uptake is less intense than on the prior scans and no new lesions are present.

Bone scan appears generally improved." In January 1993, Bruce's PSA levels had been 5.3. By March 1994, they were less than 0.3.

In July of that year, Martin Milner, N.D., medical director of the Center for Natural Medicine in Portland, Oregon, wrote, "Metastatic carcinoma of the prostate to bone has improved with objective verification on bone scan and serial PSAs with combination of orchiectomy and shark cartilage. Pain is now nonexistent."

Having scored a bull's-eye victory over his cancer, Bruce has become an outspoken advocate of shark cartilage therapy. He has won his battle; now, his mission is to see that others have the same opportunity in the war against cancer.

globe. At Shanghai Medical School in eastern China, a well-known surgeon who is also a colonel in the army is about to conduct trials involving shark cartilage's effect on liver cancer and brain cancer. Studies of shark cartilage's efficacy on breast and brain cancers are about to begin in Beijing, China, under the auspices of the Chinese National Cancer Institute. Another study in Beijing will investigate the effects of shark cartilage therapy on bone cancer. Two hospitals in Chile are currently conducting trials involving shark cartilage's effectiveness. At one hospital, children with brain tumors are receiving therapy; in the other hospital, women with breast, ovarian, or cervical cancer are receiving treatment. And in his clinic in Kyushu, Japan, Dr. Kenshi Yoshida has been studying shark cartilage's use in conjunction with immune therapy. His results have been so good (a very famous female singer in Japan has returned to her profession following treatment by Dr. Yoshida) that he has opened a clinic in Tokyo that will treat cancer patients with shark cartilage and immune therapy only.

Clinical trials in the United States and abroad will soon reveal the truth about shark cartilage's efficacy as a cancer treatment. Meanwhile, research into angiogenesis and its role in cancer and other diseases continues.

OTHER ANGIOGENESIS RESEARCH

Recently, many cancer researchers have been investigating angiogenesis's role in metastasis. Although most of this research has not involved shark cartilage, the findings help us to understand more about the probable mechanism of shark cartilage and its active proteins.

Researchers from the department of surgery at Children's Hospital in conjunction with faculty members from Harvard University and Harvard Medical School have, for instance, demonstrated that a primary tumor can stimulate angiogenesis in its own vascular bed while inhibiting the development of new blood vessels in the vascular bed of a metastasis or other secondary tumor. Inhibition and stimulation both occur in part because the angiogenesis inhibitor is retained in the circulation longer than is the angiogenesis stimulator. The researchers also reported the isolation, purification, and identification of a polypeptide (a chain of amino acids that is usually smaller than a protein) that is generated by the primary tumor and inhibits angiogenesis and growth in a secondary metastasis.

Experiments in mice demonstrated that Angiostatin, a protein that is an angiogenesis inhibitor generated by a primary tumor, can suppress growth of metastases. If the primary tumor is removed, Angiostatin levels decrease, permitting the spread of metastases. Angiostatin's ability to inhibit the growth of new blood vessels has been demonstrated for up to five days after removal of the primary tumor. The researchers believe that Angiostatin and other angiogenesis inhibitors can be very effective in the treatment of tumors. In fact, Bristol-Myers Squibb now holds exclusive worldwide licensing rights to Angiostatin, which, in preclinical trials, caused regression of primary human breast, prostate, and colon tumors in animal models. I feel confident that when work on the active proteins in shark cartilage has been completed, we will find the same active principle to be present.

Under the circumstances, it is not surprising that many researchers are now investigating agents that may halt angiogenesis. Robert Gallo, M.D., chief of the laboratory of tumor cell biology at NCI, is quoted in the March 13, 1992, issue of *Science* as saying, "Since . . . vascular proliferation, and other vascular responses are involved in a variety of pathological situations, such as tumorigenesis, inflammation and diabetic retinopathy, the development of methods to prevent or reverse their effects could have broad implications for disease treatment." At the University of Toronto, Robert S. Kerbel believes that even the effectiveness of some current anticancer drugs may rest on their antiangiogenic activity. Consider the case of interleukin-12 (IL-12).

IL-12 is known to fight cancer by activating T cells in the body's immune system. One year after clinical trials of injectible IL-12 had begun, Dr. Folkman and his associates announced that the substance also inhibited the growth of blood vessels. Scientists had noticed that the IL-12 protein inhibited dozens of different tumors in mice. Dr. Folkman and his colleagues became suspicious that IL-12 could inhibit angiogenesis because it did not destroy tumor cells in lab dishes where there is no vasculature. To test their theory, they implanted a potent inducer of blood vessel growth into mice corneas. When the IL-12 was then injected, the blood vessels stopped growing. In a subsequent test, mice that were bred to develop lung tumors received IL-12 injections. The tumors stopped growing before they had reached the size of a BB gun pellet.

There are some who even believe that an antiangiogenic agent may be the magic bullet scientists have long sought in the battle against cancer. The term "magic bullet" was actually used on the front page of a December 1994 issue of *The New York Times* when it reported on the findings of scientists at the

Scripps Research Institute in San Diego. Researchers at that institute reported finding a way to cause tumor regression with the injection of either of two proteins: a genetically engineered antibody or a synthetic peptide (molecule chain of two or more amino acids—the basic constituent of proteins). According to *The New York Times* article, these proteins inhibit the growth of blood vessels necessary for tumor growth, causing the tumors to starve and die. Experiments conducted under the leadership of Drs. David Cheresh and Peter Brooks involved grafting human cancers onto laboratory animals and then injecting the protein into the animals.

First, fragments of human tumor tissue (melanoma or lung, pancreas, and larynx carcinomas) were transplanted into ten-day old chick embryos. A day later, some of the embryos were intravenously injected with a protein (an antagonist of integrin $\alpha_v\beta_3$) and angiogenesis was disrupted, leading to regression of the transplanted tumors. Embryos that did not receive injections constituted a control group. In these embryos, blood vessels and tumors developed according to the usual patterns.

The researchers saw that the active peptide interfered with tumor-induced angiogenesis but did not affect pre-existing blood vessels. The Scripps researchers said that their findings point to an antiangiogenic therapy that may be quite powerful and made note of the fact that $\alpha_v\beta_3$ antagonists do more than prevent the growth of tumors: they actually bring about tumor regression.

Although the injected proteins elicited positive effects with a wide variety of cancers in mice, Dr. Cheresh explained that it is not known if the effects will be the same in humans. Human studies will probably not take place for at least eighteen months, at which time toxicity studies will have been completed. Various scientists warn that moving the experiments from the laboratory into clinical trials can meet with many delays.

In reporting on the research conducted by Drs. Cheresh and Brooks, a *New York Times* reporter turned to Dr. Judah Folkman,

New Hope From an Old Foe

A baby born with no arms or legs may seem like a parent's worst nightmare. But just imagine the mother's horror when she realizes her anti-morning-sickness medication was the cause of her child's deformity. Thousands of mothers—most of them in Germany—experienced this heartbreak because they had taken the drug thalidomide in their first trimester of pregnancy.

Used extensively in the 1950s to alleviate the symptoms of morning sickness and also for its sedative effects, thalidomide had always been considered a safe and effective drug. It was eventually banned in the United States when it was discovered that taking even one dose early in a pregnancy put a fetus at grave risk. Thalidomide has, however, been used continually outside the United States for the treatment of leprosy.

Now this drug, whose name once caused people to shudder, may offer hope to victims of some of the most debilitating diseases known. Scientists have discovered that the same action which puts a fetus at such risk may help to prolong life for victims of cancer and may prevent the blindness that results from diabetic retinopathy and the age-related form of macular degeneration known as "wet."

We now know that thalidomide is an antiangiogenic agent, a drug that prevents the development of new blood vessels. In an embryo, new blood vessels must form and infiltrate the limb buds or the fetus cannot develop arms and legs. Tumors also need new blood vessels to grow successfully. Without a developing network of such vessels to bring nourishment and remove waste, a tumor will die. Angiogenesis also supports the development of rheumatoid arthritis, diabetic retinopathy, and wet macular degeneration.

Thalidomide is now being used experimentally to treat cancer, rheumatoid arthritis, and macular degeneration. The National Cancer Institute plans to support five cancer trials to see whether thalidomide can stop tumor growth and even shrink tumors. Currently, research on thalidomide's effects on macular degeneration is being done at the Scheie Eye Institute in Philadelphia.

In addition to its antiangiogenic effect, thalidomide has been found to halt the replication of the HIV-1 virus in test tubes. AIDS trials are also ongoing. Researchers involved in the tests are making every effort to ensure that female subjects are not pregnant and will not become pregnant during the course of the trials.

In late December 1994—a month after shark cartilage received FDA approval for Phase II clinical trials— Science News quoted James M. Pluda, a senior investigator at NCI, as saying, "Researchers are testing other angiogenesis inhibitors as well, but only thalidomide is ready for human efficacy trials." Once again it appears that mainstream scientists will ignore a totally nontoxic natural product in favor of a pharmaceutical—even if that drug has been proven risky.

Whether thalidomide—or shark cartilage—will eventually become a standard therapy is still uncertain. But we can be sure that research into antiangiogenesis will continue until there are medications that offer real hope to victims of many diseases.

the pioneer in angiogenesis research, for a reaction to the findings. Dr. Folkman, who has always pooh-poohed shark cartilage research, expressed praise for the work conducted at Scripps. Yet shark cartilage has *already* been proven nontoxic, has been demonstrated to have antiangiogenic effects, and is already being used in humans. Here again is evidence of mainstream researchers' refusal to even consider natural products or alternative therapies.

Despite shark cartilage's promise of therapeutic efficacy, mainstream researchers continue to ignore it while pursuing tortuous research paths. At Northwestern University's biochemistry department and in its medical school, for instance, researchers are investigating two proteins synthesized in the placenta. One of these proteins has been found to stimulate endothelial cell migration in cultures and the growth of new blood vessels in vivo, and the other inhibits these activities. The researchers can only conclude that the protein known as placental proliferin (PLF) *may* play a role in certain tumors.

Other research on angiogenesis is being conducted at Northwestern University Medical School and the University of Texas M.D. Anderson Cancer Center in Houston. In a 1994 article in *Science*, scientists there reported having found a genetically controlled mechanism that decreases the levels of thrombospondin, which normally binds to the cells that form blood vessels. Without thrombospondin, these cells cannot grow into new blood vessels. According to one of the participants in the study, there is hope that thrombospondin and other naturally occurring proteins will eventually develop into nontoxic drugs that can effectively stop the growth of small tumors.

The search for such drugs is, in fact, so intense that at least eight companies are currently conducting clinical trials of drugs that can starve rather than kill cancer cells. We know all too well that killing cancer cells often destroys healthy tissues. Therapies that rely on antiangiogenesis interfere with the creation of new blood vessels without harming healthy tissue. And cancer cells will probably not become resistant to antiangiogenic agents. Whereas cancer cells often become resistant to chemotherapy because they mutate, the genes found in the endothelial cells of developing blood vessels are very stable. No wonder the search for a marketable angiogenesis inhibitor has become so popular. Believing that antiangiogenesis is the key to a revolution in cancer therapy, mainstream scientists are testing such antiangiogenic agents as platelet factor 4, cartilage-derived inhibitor (CDI—what shark cartilage is), and a fungal product and its analog (a substance functionally similar but structurally different from the fungal product).

Daiichi Pharmaceutical, a Japanese company, is currently

conducting research into SP-PG (sulfated polysaccharide-peptidoglycan), a carbohydrate produced by a bacterium. This carbohydrate has been shown to inhibit growth of vascular endothelial cells in vitro. Although not yet purified, the most active fraction inhibits the growth of experimental solid tumors that require angiogenesis for their growth. One experiment involved Kaposi's sarcoma (KS).

AIDS-KS cells induce blood vessel development in chicken chorioallantoic membranes (CAM); when transplanted into nude mice, the cells cause leaking of blood vessels, edema (swelling), angiogenesis, and the development of KS-like lesions. SP-PG inhibited the development of new blood vessels. It also inhibited the vascular leaking and angiogenesis associated with the introduction of AIDS-KS cells into nude mice.

The present study suggests that SP-PG may be promising as a therapy for Kaposi's sarcoma, which is characterized by angiogenesis in the first stage of lesion development. SP-PG has little toxicity and limits the growth of AIDS-KS cells and the development of KS-like lesions. The cytotoxic agent pentosan polysulfate, which is currently being used as KS therapy, has not inhibited the development of angiogenic lesions.

Dr. Folkman and his colleagues are also conducting experiments with a chemical found in a particular fungus. This chemical (AGM-1470) has been shown to inhibit the growth of certain melanomas. It is now undergoing clinical trials (see *The Japanese Connection* beginning on page 76).

As reported in the *Journal of the National Cancer Institute* in February 1994, tissue inhibitor metalloproteinase (TIMP-2) is a protein that "is known to inhibit tumor invasion and metastasis." The amino acid sequences or protein structure of TIMP-2 is similar to that found in cartilage-derived inhibitor (CDI).

William G. Stetler-Stevenson, M.D., of the National Institutes of Health and his co-workers report in the February 2, 1994 *Journal of the National Cancer Institute* that TIMP-2's ability to block the migration and proliferation of cells is similar to that

Metastasis—The Real Killer

*The diagnosis of a tumor is not a death sentence. Far from it. Many tumors are benign, little more than abnormal swellings. In fact, **tumor** is the Latin word for "swelling." And even if a tumor is malignant—growing uncontrollably—removing or killing the tumor can be completely successful.*

In actuality, more patients die as a result of metastasis—the spread of cancer cells from one site to another—than from original or primary tumors. A tumor can cause death only if it becomes so large that it chokes off a vital organ, such as the lungs or liver. If a tumor is malignant, however, it has the potential for metastasis.

When cancer is metastatic, abnormal tissue growth appears in parts of the body that are remote from the primary tumor. Metastasis occurs when cancer cells travel to other places in the body through the blood and/or lymphatic vessels. Metastasis is not, however, a foregone conclusion. In many cases, tumor cells become trapped in the small capillaries or venules. In other cases, traveling tumor cells are destroyed by the body's defense mechanisms or by unfavorable conditions in the environment such as insufficient nutrients.

When tumor cells break off from the tumor and are not stopped, they travel through the blood or lymph system into the first available downward-flowing capillary bed or lymph node. The lung is a common site for metastasis because the heart pumps blood through the pulmonary vessels before it goes anywhere else. The liver is also a common site for intestinal cancers to metastasize because the liver gets some of its blood from the intestines.

Metastatic cells are usually different from the original tumor cells. They undergo mutations in order to dislodge and begin a new colony. Sometimes these colonies have a more heterogeneous or diverse population that can make them more resistant to therapy. And oftentimes, it is impossible to find all of the secondary tumors that result from metastasis. Chemotherapy then becomes the best if not only treatment option.

> *Conventional treatment strategies call for the surgical re-moval of tumors or tumor destruction with radiation and/or chemotherapy. The best defense against metastasis is to destroy the tumor before metastasis can begin.*

of CDI. Not only does TIMP-2 block cell invasion, but it also blocks tumor growth. Dr. Stetler-Stevenson has said that TIMP-2 might inhibit angiogenesis. He believes that TIMP and CDI may be a lot more similar than once thought and writes in the same article that TIMP might be the active component of carti-lage, giving it anti-metastatic properties. TIMP-2 is now under-going clinical trials and Dr. Stetler-Stevenson believes that if progress continues, antiangiogenic drugs may be powerful can-cer treatments in the future. But, like Drs. Langer and Folkman, Dr. Stetler-Stevenson believes that administering shark carti-lage orally or by injection would probably preclude the ab-sorbtion of TIMP-2 if it were present. Yet we have seen that numerous proteins are absorbed when administered by these routes. The search for a marketable angiogenesis inhibitor is also being conducted in California.

One Researcher's Quest

Kin-Ping Wong, Ph.D., known as "K.P.," is dean of the School of Natural Sciences at Fresno State University in Fresno, Cali-fornia. He has been involved in the field of protein synthesis for more than twenty years; for the last ten, he has been working to isolate the active components in shark cartilage. Formerly a professor and dean at the University of Kansas and a National Science Foundation (NSF) researcher, Dr. Wong vigorously pursued basic research into protein synthesis. Eventually, he wanted to be involved in research that could be applied to helping people, research out of which he could "get more satisfaction." Looking for an area in which he could make a contribution, Dr. Wong was quick to discern that cancer was "one of the most challenging areas." He was concerned that the traditional ways of dealing with cancer were so toxic. He believed that with all of the recent developments in biochemistry, there had to be other ways of treating this disease.

Dr. Wong began to read about the latest developments in cancer research and soon stumbled across an article written by an eye doctor for a journal so obscure that he no longer remembers its name. The eye doctor had written that the critical stage in the development of cancer is the period in which neovascularization (formation of new blood vessels) occurs near the tumor, which Dr. Wong says, ". . . is obvious to everyone now. We know that once vascularization occurs, the tumor grows very fast." Dr. Wong then read about Dr. Langer's work at MIT, in which an extract of shark cartilage was implanted near tumors in the eyes of rabbits, and the tumors largely stopped growing (see page 9).

The issue of neovascularization—angiogenesis—soon occupied Dr. Wong's thoughts, and he began discussing the topic with a former student, Carl Leur, Ph.D. A marine biologist, Dr. Leur had gotten an NSF grant to study sharks, particularly their resistance to toxic materials. On a visit to Dr. Leur's Florida lab, Dr. Wong learned that sharks rarely get cancer although other marine animals often die of the disease. Out of thousands of autopsies conducted on sharks, there have been only a dozen or so proven cases of cancer. When Dr. Leur told Dr. Wong that sharks were composed almost entirely of cartilage, Dr. Wong visualized unchartered territory that he could explore in the pursuit of knowledge and satisfaction.

"As a biochemist," says Dr. Wong, "I believed from the start that there is a chemical substance in the shark that inhibits the growth of capillaries. In biological systems, if something promotes growth, something else inhibits it or it will run out of control." (This theory has now been proven by Dr. Folkman.) Determined to identify that substance, Dr. Wong began his quest as any traditional scientist does: he wrote a grant proposal. Recognizing the waste involved in selling shark steaks, but throwing away the cartilage, the Department of Commerce awarded Dr. Wong a National Sea Grant. Dr. Wong started working with six graduate students and an equal number of technicians. Although his work at first involved measuring inhibition of vascularization with the CAM assay, he found that technique to be too subjective. He has now developed a cell culture technique that he believes will "become the standard for measuring inhibition of capillary growth."

In this new technique, Dr. Wong cultures or grows the cells that make up the lining of blood vessels. He then exposes these endothelial cells to a variety of substances and determines which substances inhibit replication of the cells. If the cells do not reproduce, new blood vessels do not form. Through the use of these tests, Dr. Wong has been able to isolate several proteins in shark cartilage that are antiangiogenic.

Although he has received some media attention, Dr. Wong is reluctant to say too much about his work; he is currently trying to obtain patents and there are private investors interested in the research. He does say that he is now culturing cartilage cells in order to obtain the angiogenesis inhibitor from the culture media. Dr. Wong and his associates believe the inhibitor holds great promise as a treatment for cancer. He hopes that with a patent and private funding, there may someday be a marketable product.

IN CONCLUSION

There are many physicians and researchers who would like to go on discussing how much of the active protein found in shark cartilage is absorbed. They remind me of the story about ancient philosophers who debated how many angels can fit on the head of a pin. The critical aspect of the shark cartilage debate, however, is not philosophy or theory but practicality.

Physicians all over the world have been using whole shark cartilage on patients and have been getting results. The response appears to be there and appears to be fairly consistent. We're getting a positive response in 60 to 70 percent of the cases. Discussion of theories is great, but results are all that really matter. When you're dealing with terminal patients, when hope is minimal, and when you have a natural product that is nontoxic, why wait until you do forty years of research, and 20 million people die? Continue the research, but get the results with the people, the victims.

How much protein is getting through—10 percent, 40 percent, 90 percent? I don't know, but *enough* is getting through to give us results. And I really believe that the name of the game is not theory but clinical results. The reactions of sick people are more important than slow ruminations over possibilities.

Although we are not now certain of the mechanism(s) involved, we are certain of the results we are seeing over and over again. Patients taking shark cartilage are experiencing shrinkage of tumor size, decrease in pain, and an overall increase in their quality of life. Doctors all over the world are admitting conventional options often fail. Read the words of a report in *Science* in March 1995:

> But the triumphs so far have led only to sporadic successes in the clinic. While death rates for some cancers have declined, others have increased, particularly among older people.

Shark cartilage is, indeed, an option that appears very exciting.

At the end of the symposium he moderated at Metropolitan Hospital Center (see page 83), Dr. Holt said, "Can we leave here with the message that shark cartilage is the panacea for cancer? Of course not. But we have a very clear indication that there is some beneficial effect observed at the clinical level that requires at least careful scrutiny to give us another option in disorders where we have few options."

Someday, all of the mechanisms will be understood. Someday, the active protein(s) will be isolated, purified, and synthesized. Today, come learn with us as we work with those who have, until now, had no hope. Today, come rejoice with those who have found hope.

8.

Arthritis Studies

In its various forms, arthritis disables more people than any other chronic disorder.

The New Columbia Encyclopedia

Of all the "ills that man is heir to" perhaps the most perplexing are the autoimmune diseases in which the body's defense system actually attacks the body. The most infamous of the autoimmune conditions is AIDS (acquired immune deficiency syndrome), and one of the most common is arthritis.

While cancer annually afflicts over 1 million new people in the United States alone, arthritis (inflammation of the joints) is considered the most common debilitating disorder in the temperate areas of the world; 50 million people—including 200,000 children—suffer from one of more than one hundred forms. The disorder is so common that fossil evidence indicates prehistoric people and even dinosaurs suffered from it. In the United States in the twentieth century, 13 million people seek medical treatment for arthritis each year. More than 750,000 of these people cannot function sufficiently well to perform daily tasks.

THE ARTHRITIS PICTURE TODAY

The term *arthritis* refers to any inflammation of the joints. There are numerous forms of the condition, some of which—like acute pyogenic arthritis and septic arthritis—are bacterial in origin. Less is known, however, about the origins of the most common forms of arthritis—osteoarthritis (OA) and rheumatoid arthritis (RA).

Osteoarthritis, or osteoarthrosis, is a destructive disease of the cartilage in joints (articular cartilage). It is the most prevalent rheumatic disorder in the world; 40 million people suffer from it in the United States alone. Often considered a disease of aging, osteoarthritis is marked by changes in joint tissues. Joints in a young person are cushioned and lubricated by cartilage pads and synovial membranes. As time goes on, the cartilage and smooth membranes become eroded. OA may also result, at least in part, from an immune system response. Cartilage that normally cushions the joint becomes soft and breaks down. Small pieces of bone and cartilage become loose and are caught inside the joint. The body's immune system may interpret the fragments as injury and, in response, generate inflammation at the site, causing pain.

Almost everyone over the age of fifty has at least the beginning signs of osteoarthritis, but rheumatoid arthritis usually strikes those under the age of forty-five. A systemic disorder that causes a thickening of the soft tissue and erosion of cartilage in joints, rheumatoid arthritis tends to be chronic and progressive, resulting ultimately in deformities and disability. It is believed that rheumatoid arthritis is an autoimmune disease in which small circulating white blood cells (T cells) react to an apparently foreign body (antigen) within the joint. It is possible that type II collagen, a protein common in joint cartilage, may be the target of the autoimmune response; antigens normally are proteins. The immune response causes inflammation, which results in pain.

Arthritis may also be an angiogenesis-dependent disease.

In people with arthritis, the synovial fluid that lubricates joint cartilage contains a compound that stimulates the growth of blood vessels. Called endothelial cell stimulating angiogenesis factor or ESAF, it precipitates the invasion of blood vessels into cartilage, which leads to calcification. Remember, in the embryo, capillaries invade cartilage as the preliminary step in bone development. It is not surprising that recent studies supported by the National Institutes of Health lead to the conclusion that angiogenesis is an important factor in inflammatory disorders such as rheumatoid arthritis.

There are no treatments available to control osteoarthritis or rheumatoid arthritis, or to correct damage caused by these diseases. Current treatments are limited to control of pain and inflammation. To date, one of the most effective means of controlling the inflammation and associated pain has been the use of steroids, naturally occurring fat-soluble compounds.

Steroids have certainly received their fair share of "bad press." We have all heard of athletes—even Olympic contenders—who have put their physical health and reputations at risk because of steroid use. Those with arthritis, Lupus, and some other chronic diseases may not fear a loss of reputation but are rightfully terrified of the well-publicized harmful side effects of the drugs. These people must choose between the debilitating effects of their disease and the potential of stomach irritation, glaucoma, and decreased immune system function that occurs with high doses or prolonged use of steroids.

The risk of incurring the harmful side effects from steroid use is lifelong because symptomatic relief is obtained only so long as the drugs are taken. Unfortunately, withdrawal from the drugs can cause severe recurrence of the original symptoms. Even the nonsteroidal anti-inflammatory drugs (NSAIDS) such as aspirin have a host of potentially serious side effects—ulcers, buzzing in the ears, damage to the intestinal lining, and intestinal bleeding.

Surgery—complete or partial prosthetic replacement—produces the most rapid and dramatic improvements for victims of severe arthritis. More than 600 thousand knees, hips, and shoulders are replaced annually. In fact, I have had an artificial hip for more than twenty years—the result of a serious automobile accident in Africa. Fortunately, it works well and I have been pain-free for all these years.

But joint replacements are costly, use valuable resources, and are not always totally successful. They also carry an inherent risk of infection and mortality, particularly in the elderly. The risks and costs are, of course, multiplied when a patient is affected in several major joints. In an effort to reduce at least some of these negative factors, the possibility of replacing damaged cartilage naturally rather than prosthetically is currently being investigated.

Orthopedic researcher Daniel Grane at North Shore University Hospital/New York University Medical Center cultured sheets of cartilage-secreting cells called chondrocytes in enough quantity to resurface the injured knee joints of rabbits and dogs. Subsequently, a bio-tech company in Massachusetts received a patent on a process for cloning healthy new cartilage tissue from cells taken from damaged cartilage. In 1995, approximately sixty patients in the United States were able to have their knee cartilage replaced because of this process. In a three-step procedure that costs between $20 and $25,000, the patients first underwent arthroscopic surgery to remove damaged cartilage cells, which were then used to clone new cartilage. During a second surgical procedure, a small incision was made in the person's shin and a piece of periosteum (the thin tissue covering the bone) was removed. A six-inch incision was made in the knee, the periosteum was sutured over the area, and the cloned tissue was inserted. The patients then underwent a four-to-six month period of rehabilitation. At this time, the technique is being used to treat injuries to knee cartilage only. Physicians hope that early treatment can prevent the onset of osteoarthritis.

Presently, there is not much that can be done for those with arthritis. In fact, the prognosis for arthritis sufferers has always been so dismal that the *Medical and Health Encyclopedia* offers this advice:

> The arthritis patient needs to develop a sense of coexistence with the disease, a tolerant attitude toward the problem of possible pain or disability without surrendering to arthritis. Millions of people have learned to live with arthritis.

It is no wonder that the search is on to find drugs that can reduce the inflammation responsible for pain without producing negative side effects. Researchers at Texas A&M University's Health Science Center report they may have found a synthetic version of the substances that control inflammation as part of the body's immune response to injury. The substance is a laboratory-produced version of what is called interleukin-1 blockers, which occur naturally in the human body and are produced by the immune system in response to injury or infection. Dr. George C.Y. Chiou, one of the A&M researchers, points out that there isn't a single preparation that begins to approach the steroids in effectiveness. And the synthetic substances he is working with are about seven times as effective as the steroid prednisolone.

The ideal arthritis medication would reduce inflammation by a disease-specific mechanism with no toxic side effects. Antiangiogenic substances such as shark cartilage are one promising avenue of research.

ANTIANGIOGENESIS OFFERS THERAPEUTIC POSSIBILITIES

The concept of using cartilage to treat arthritis is not restricted to proponents of alternative medicine. To my knowledge, the first person to use cartilage as an arthritis treatment was Harvard-trained surgeon Dr. John Prudden over twenty-five years ago. More recently, a group of Harvard researchers turned their attention to the use of chicken cartilage as an arthritis therapy (see page 137). But we should not make light of the work of Dr. Prudden, who pioneered medicinal uses for cartilage.

Early experiments conducted by Dr. Prudden indicated that a cartilage-derived angiogenesis inhibitor had a beneficial effect on arthritis. In a study involving nine people aged forty-three through sixty-nine who suffered from severe rheumatoid arthritis, Dr. Prudden found that a dose of 500 cc of bovine cartilage subcutaneously administered for ten to thirty-five days and followed by booster doses at three- to four-week intervals as needed, elicited "astonishingly good" results. Evaluations of those in the study showed arthritic conditions going from "severe" to either "excellent" or "good."

In a subsequent study conducted by Dr. Prudden, twenty-eight arthritic patients, all with severe pain and major functional disability, were injected with a cartilage preparation over a period of three to eight weeks. Twenty-five of the patients showed good to excellent improvement.

In the early 1980s, other studies using bovine cartilage were conducted on arthritis sufferers in clinics in five Eastern European countries. The most significant aspect of these studies was the data on lost working days. Over a 10-year period, patients receiving a bovine cartilage preparation lost an average of just 20 working days per year; the patients who did not receive the cartilage preparation lost a steadily increasing number of working days, culminating in a total of 180 out of 250 days by the tenth year of the study. The pain associated with arthritis was decreased by 85 percent when cartilage was administered; patients in the control group used nonsteroidal anti-inflammatory drugs or placebos and experienced only a 5 percent reduction in pain. Joint degeneration among those using the cartilage amounted to only 37 percent of the control group's joint degeneration.

In 1987, the results of a long-term assessment of the effects of a bovine cartilage preparation on osteoarthritis were published by the head of the rheumatology facility at Charles University in Prague, Czechoslovakia. This was a double-blind study, which meant that neither the 194 participating patients nor the doctors knew who was getting the cartilage material and who was getting the placebo. When patients were "scored" according to their levels of pain, pain scores dropped an average of 50 percent.

One of the earliest studies using shark cartilage was conducted by Dr. Serge Orloff, a leading arthritis expert in Western Europe. He administered some of the earliest dried shark cartilage I had prepared. (It was encapsulated in my kitchen with the assistance of Eva Gottscho, who has helped me with my work for years.) Dr. Orloff gave his patients 9 grams of cartilage daily for four weeks, followed by 4.5 grams daily for two weeks, and was impressed with the results.

In 1989, José A. Orcasita, M.D., then assistant clinical professor of internal medicine at the University of Miami School of Medicine and now in private practice in Miami Lakes, conducted a nine-week study of the effects of oral administration of shark cartilage on three elderly victims of osteoarthritis. In all cases, the patients showed a marked improvement in their quality of life. In the same year, Dr. Carlos Luis Alpizar, head of the national geriatric program in Costa Rica, gave daily oral doses of shark cartilage to ten patients suffering from such severe osteoarthritis that they were bedridden. Within three weeks, eight of the patients were ambulatory. To ensure that the positive results from shark cartilage were not due to a placebo effect—a psychological rather than a real effect—a veterinarian in Brussels, Belgium, conducted a carefully controlled study with dogs. Jacques Rauis, D.V.M., a member of the faculty of medicine at the University of Liege, reported on his study at the 1991 Small Animal Veterinary Congress in Manchester, England.

Dr. Rauis's studies were conducted using dried shark cartilage, which I had prepared, as treatment for secondary

Bovine Cartilage versus Shark Cartilage

The earliest human studies involving cartilage therapy were conducted in the 1960s. At that time, it was found that bovine cartilage could be used to accelerate wound healing. Recently, there has been renewed interest in bovine cartilage, generated at least in part by a growing interest in natural remedies in general and shark cartilage in particular. This interest is being further fueled by a public relations firm in the Midwest.

Publicity generated by this company claims the activity of shark cartilage is derived primarily from mucopolysaccharides and that bovine cartilage is more effective. While it is true that bovine cartilage contains more mucopolysaccharides than shark cartilage—a fact I often mention—I strongly believe that properly processed shark cartilage is materially more effective in cancerous tumors than is bovine cartilage. Just because both are cartilage does not mean they are basically the same. Oranges and apples are both fruit, but they are vastly different. And shark cartilage differs vastly from bovine cartilage in its mechanism of action.

Along with mucopolysaccharides, shark cartilage contains active proteins that inhibit angiogenesis. Bovine cartilage has far less antiangiogenic effect—approximately 1,000 times less as demonstrated by Drs. Langer and Lee at MIT (see page 9). In the processing of bovine cartilage, acetone is used to remove the fat that clings to the cartilage. This procedure denatures (renders inactive) the proteins responsible for angiogenesis. Since there is no fat on shark cartilage, the processing procedure is less likely to denature the active proteins. In other words, bovine cartilage has little antiangiogenic effect; its therapeutic value stems from the mucopolysaccharides' ability to stimulate the immune system. When advanced, nonresponsive cancer patients show improvement during shark cartilage therapy, it is the antiangiogenic action of the proteins that is the pivotal factor.

Consider the most recent results of trials using bovine cartilage as a cancer therapy. One company involved in research and
development of a bovine cartilage product received an IND in the
mid-1980s and began conducting clinical trials using an inject-
able form of the bovine cartilage. A Securities and Exchange
Commission (SEC) filing made by the company in 1994 docu-
ments the results of four clinical trials. Twenty-five solid-tumor
patients participated in the first two studies of safety and preliminary efficacy conducted in Newark, New Jersey, and Her-
shey, Pennsylvania. Only one of these patients had a complete
remission. Twenty-four of the patients died.

Phase II trials to determine bovine cartilage's efficacy for
specific conditions as well as dosage and possible side effects are
currently being conducted in Montreal, Canada, and Westchester,
New York. These trials involve forty-six patients with kidney
cancer. According to Dr. Carmelo Puccio, M.D., principal investigator for the trials being conducted at Westchester County
Medical Center, two patients have experienced partial remission:
one over a period of two and a half years, and one over several
months. Another patient has experienced complete remission
after four years.

In short, out of the seventy-one patients involved in the
bovine cartilage trials, only four (5.6 percent) have experienced
significant change in their disease states. On the other hand,
when properly processed shark cartilage has been administered
to cancer patients, we have seen tumor shrinkage in better than
50 percent of the cases.

Publicity and marketing campaigns for bovine cartilage
products have focused on only the small percentage of patients
that showed any response to the material. This emphasis makes
it seem as though a significant result has been achieved when, in
fact, little effect was demonstrated.

I also take exception to the claims that 9 grams of orally
administered bovine cartilage have the same effect as higher shark
cartilage doses. The studies used to substantiate these claims were
conducted largely with an "injected" suspension of bovine cartilage.

(A few of the subjects received a combination of both oral and injected.) Absorption of orally and intravenously administered substances is quite different. Without research based on oral administration, it is really not possible to gauge—or compare— appropriate oral dosage.

And what of the claim that bovine cartilage is more effective than shark cartilage because it has a higher percentage of mu- copolysaccharides? As far as I know, there has been no assay for mucopolysaccharides; in fact, carbohydrate content is often de- termined by adding up the other known components of a sub- stance and then subtracting that total from 100 percent; the remainder is considered to be carbohydrate.

Furthermore, the first human study with shark cartilage employed a product made from shark fin fibers. This product (prohibitively expensive as a commercial preparation) was about 92 percent protein. When you consider that moisture accounted for approximately 7 percent, there were basically very few mu- copolysaccharides in the product. When this almost pure-protein shark cartilage was tested in Mexico, we got the best results ever obtained: seven of eight cancer patients survived; five of the seven were basically tumor free; two had 80 percent tumor reduction in just eleven weeks. Obviously, the lack of mucopolysac- charides was not detrimental to the product's effectiveness.

Both shark and bovine cartilage products have their uses. For osteoarthritis by itself, bovine cartilage may be more effective than shark cartilage. However, for the other angiogenic diseases such as rheumatoid arthritis, psoriasis, and diabetic retinopathy, shark cartilage is theoretically superior.

I believe that bovine cartilage does stimulate the immune system, but for patients suffering from diseases related to angio- genesis, shark—not bovine—cartilage is the therapy of choice. Positive therapeutic results obtained with shark cartilage are based on angiogenesis inhibition and product activity, not on carbohydrate activity. Immune stimulation is important, but it is the active proteins that are the key to shark cartilage's effec- tiveness.

osteoarthritis in ten dogs, each of whom suffered from severe lameness. The dogs were periodically evaluated both during and after the treatment. Dr. Rauis quickly found dramatic decreases in the signs of the disease. In eight of the ten dogs, lameness disappeared and the animals' capacity for getting around obstacles improved tremendously. Swelling, pain, and immobilization were negligible. When the cartilage was discontinued after twenty-one days of treatment, most of the dogs reverted in large part to their original pained state within fifteen days. When the shark cartilage was again added to their diet, the improvement seemed to be even better, occurred more quickly than originally, and was achieved with 50 percent of the original dosage level. (Subsequently, another six dogs were studied with similar results.) The dog studies confirm the results that have been achieved in humans and eliminate the possibility that the effect is psychological rather than physiological.

And in Panama, Harry X. Andres, M.D., has also been investigating the effects of shark cartilage on arthritis with excellent—although limited—results. In Cuba during the clinical trials to determine shark cartilage's efficacy as a cancer treatment (see pages 95–98), physicians noted that in patients with rheumatoid arthritis as well as psoriasis, these conditions improved or even disappeared after three to five weeks. Both rheumatoid arthritis and psoriasis are fairly common in advanced cancer patients, possibly because both chemotherapy and radiation reduce the activity of the immune system. The high dosage level of shark cartilage used in the Cuban trial has led me to suggest a moderately high dosage (30 to 40 grams per day) for psoriasis and rheumatoid arthritis patients, who have been reporting unusually good results.

Considering the components of shark cartilage, it is not really surprising that the cartilage is effective for arthritis sufferers. The mucopolysaccharides in shark cartilage seem to fight inflammation. The complex carbohydrates found in the cartilage—particularly chondroitin sulphate A and C—have long been used in the safe and effective treatment of chronic inflammatory diseases. Furthermore, proteins in shark cartilage appear to block the angiogenic process, which is now known to be associated with the development of arthritis.

It has been established that tumor necrosis factor (TNF) plays a major role in the pathogenesis of rheumatoid arthritis. TNF has been shown to induce erosion of both cartilage and bone. When, for instance, TNF was introduced into the cartilage in rabbits' knees, cartilage injury ensued. An extensive report of the relationship between TNF and rheumatoid arthritis appeared in the October 1992 journal *Arthritis and Rheumatism.* The authors report that in rheumatoid arthritis TNF was detectable in up to 90 percent of the cells in the synovial lining and was found in vascular endothelial cells, the activity of which has a direct role in angiogenesis. TNF was also found in osteoarthritic synovia and in normal synovial tissue but in much lesser quantities. The TNF was most evident where there was tissue destruction. Because TNF, a known angiogenesis-inducer, has now been conclusively implicated in rheumatoid arthritis, it would appear that an angiogenesis-inhibitor could be effective in arthritis therapy. Recent research out of Harvard indicates that the inhibitor may indeed be present in shark cartilage.

FURTHER STUDIES

Research into cartilage involves more than the study of antiangiogenesis. Research conducted by David Trentham, M.D., a rheumatologist (a physician who treats diseases of the muscles, tendons, joints, bones, or nerves that result in discomfort and disability) at Harvard, indicates that more than the antiangiogenic characteristics and the mucopolysaccharides in shark cartilage may be involved in arthritis relief.

In the study conducted by Dr. Trentham, patients with severe rheumatoid arthritis received oral doses of type II collagen obtained from chicken cartilage. Use of an orally ingested protein to combat disease is based on the body's ability to ingest the protein in foods without incurring immune reactions. This process, called *oral tolerization*, occurs when foreign proteins enter the body through the digestive system and suppress immune responses rather than trigger them. A therapeutic use of the system was first tried in humans suffering from multiple sclerosis who were fed myelin, a brain substance. Now collagen—the protein found at the site of the autoimmune disease—has been fed to arthritis patients in the hopes that ingesting the collagen may trigger the autoimmunity initially, subsequently reducing autoimmune attacks.

In the first trial conducted by Dr. Trentham, ten arthritis patients were taken off all drugs and given 0.1 mg of solubilized type II collagen daily for one month, followed by 0.5 mg for two months. One of the ten patients experienced a complete remission that continued for twenty-six months. Six of the subjects experienced a "substantial clinical response," an improvement of 50 percent or more in joint swelling and tenderness combined with improvement of 50 percent in two of the following disease measures: morning stiffness, walk time, grip strength, erythrocyte sedimentation rate (the speed with which the red blood cells fall to the bottom of a test tube is a measure of inflammation), or global assessments by physician or patient. The improvement had to last for at least two months after treatment. None of the patients experienced side effects. Four patients had relapses approximately three months after the therapy concluded but experienced benefits when the collagen therapy was reinitiated. According to the researchers involved in the study, "These data demonstrate clinical efficacy of an oral tolerization approach for rheumatoid arthritis."

In a subsequent double-blind trial (neither patients nor researchers know whether the therapeutic agent or a placebo is being administered), sixty patients ceased taking their immunosuppressive drugs. About half the study subjects received the same collagen dose as in the first trial, and the other half were given a placebo, which was taken orally for ninety consecutive days. Both groups had similar demographic, clinical, and laboratory parameters. Patients in the collagen group exhibited significant improvement in the number of swollen joints, number of tender or painful joints, and walk-time in the first, second, and third months. Overall, this group had a 25 to 30 percent reduction in observed swelling. Those patients in the placebo group, who were now off their immonosuppressive drugs, actually tended to deteriorate. For those in the collagen group, no side effects were evident nor were there significant changes in laboratory values. The researchers concluded that the controlled trial is evidence that oral administration of small quantities of type II collagen is safe and can improve clinical signs of active rheumatoid arthritis. The trials imply that an orally administered protein can, according to the September 29, 1993 *Science* article, "down-regulate specific autoimmune disease as long as it is a constituent of the target tissue and is capable of inducing regulatory T cells."

We know that shark cartilage contains a number of active proteins, and it is reasonable to assume that one or more of these proteins also occurs in human cartilage. Also, if collagen—a major constituent of cartilage—is effective as an arthritis therapy, cartilage should be too. Dr. Trentham's work indicates to me that it is theoretically possible that oral administration of shark cartilage can have a therapeutic effect on an autoimmune disease such as arthritis. Equally important, his work demonstrates that orally ingested proteins can find their way into the bloodstream in a biologically active form.

Dr. Trentham's work with chicken cartilage was proclaimed a "breakthrough" by many media representatives, but shark cartilage's effects on arthritis have rarely been mentioned in the media. Because the work on chicken cartilage comes from within the medical establishment, it is okay to say that the use of that cartilage holds promise for relief of arthritic pain.

IN CONCLUSION

Although the studies of shark cartilage as an arthritis therapy are limited, the results are promising. Current theories indicating that arthritis is an angiogenesis-dependent disease imply that shark cartilage should be an effective therapeutic agent. Furthermore, physicians currently administering shark cartilage to arthritis patients orally or rectally (see page 150 for specific instructions) note that administration of 8 to 15 grams on a daily basis materially improves the condition.

In the words of V. Rejholee, M.D., published in *Seminars in Arthritis and Rheumatism* in 1987:

> It is clear that any form of medication that is well tolerated and shown to be capable of . . . either slowing progression or by bringing about actual regression, must be regarded as a major advance in the therapy for this condition. The implications in terms of relief of suffering, health care resources and socioeconomic costs to the community are similarly far reaching. Therefore, any therapeutic agent with indications of such activity must be considered and carefully evaluated.

I think the good doctor made his point well.

9.

Administration of Shark Cartilage

With little new ground gained in the war against cancer, no cure in sight for AIDS, and the looming threat of resistance to current antibiotics, modern researchers have become as intrigued by new natural pharmaceuticals as 15th-century explorers were by spices.

Faye Flam
Science

Ll around the world—in Canada, the United States, Brazil, Hungary, Israel, Japan, Korea, China, Spain, Australia, Great Britain—people are using shark cartilage as a therapeutic agent for some types of cancer, arthritis, macular degeneration, and other diseases, as well as a prophylactic against them. Almost daily, I am bombarded by questions: How much shark cartilage should I take? How often should I take it? Does it matter which brand I use?

People who use or want to use shark cartilage as a therapeutic or prophylactic agent must understand that there are—as yet—no concrete answers to these questions. All we now have are the observations made in the field.

DOSAGE IS DERIVED FROM EXPERIENCE

Researchers have administered whole shark cartilage to cancer patients participating in clinical trials and have, in many cases, seen outstanding results. Physicians have worked with cancer patients who use shark cartilage, sometimes advising them about dosage and sometimes simply monitoring the patients' progress while they were taking the cartilage. The researchers and physicians have observed the dosages that appear to be optimal, and their observations are noted here.

In all of the clinical trials, a dosage of 1 gram of shark cartilage per kilogram (2.2 pounds) of body weight has been used on a daily basis with promising results. (These trials used a cartilage material averaging around 35 percent protein.) For example, a person who weighs 150 pounds would take an average of 68 grams of the cartilage daily. With patients who have very serious tumors—such as liver, kidney, or pancreatic—or very advanced malignancies, higher doses are sometimes used. In these cases, physicians have administered as much as 2 grams of similar material per kilogram of body weight with good responses and no side effects. Lately, with a new shark cartilage product containing an average of 42 percent protein, the average dose is being reduced accordingly.

Shark cartilage comes in two forms—pills and loose powder. Because taking 100 or more pills daily is difficult, most people are using the cartilage in its powdered form. The powdered cartilage can be taken either orally or rectally. (In all current clinical trials, in both the United States and abroad, cartilage is being administered orally.) When preparing the powder for oral consumption, patients mix up to 20 grams (four level teaspoons) with six to eight ounces of a vegetable juice such as tomato or carrot, or a fruit nectar such as pineapple or apricot, in a blender to produce a frothy shake. They then drink these shakes three to four times daily, usually thirty minutes before meals. When taken on an empty stomach, the drink passes rapidly through the stomach acids, avoiding breakdown of the active proteins. Doses are best taken throughout the day to maintain a fairly constant level of active protein in the blood.

Several physicians, such as Neal Adelman, M.D., of Short Hills, New Jersey, have found the above-mentioned method of oral consumption to be effective. His patients use a blender to mix small doses (10 to 15 grams) of the cartilage powder. They drink the mixture four to six times a day and have shown no stomach upset, little resistance, and very good responses. Dr. Adelman and Dr. Donald Angeliti of West Caldwell, New Jersey, normally start their patients with 1 gram of cartilage per kilogram of body weight, increasing the dosage to 1½ to 2 grams within the first two weeks.

At first, it had appeared that rectal administration of the powdered cartilage was superior to oral. Today, all feel that oral or rectal administration is equally effective. The FDA trials currently underway are all based on oral administration. Although most patients prefer taking the product orally, some simply cannot. Some people have intestinal reactions to ingested cartilage, still others, due to nausea or esophogeal blockages, may be unable to hold down the oral dose. These people are taking the cartilage rectally.

When shark cartilage is administered rectally, a retention enema is prepared consisting of a well-mixed solution of 20 grams of powdered shark cartilage in three to four ounces of body-temperature water. A few drops of aloe vera (the juice or gel obtained from the leaves of the succulent plant of the same name and sold in health food stores) may be added to produce a smoother mix.

In order to introduce this water-suspension solution into the rectal area, the following things are needed: a small piece (6 to 8 inches) of hose from a standard enema bag and three to four 60 to 80 cc syringes. Administration of the dosage is quite simple. First, the syringes are loaded with the cartilage solution. One end of the hose is then inserted into the rectum. The tip of one of the filled syringes is next placed in the other end of the hose. The solution is pushed through the tube into the rectum, using one syringe at a time. The patient then lies on his or her right side for twenty-five minutes to facilitate retention, and thereby, absorption. (When a person lies on the right side, the solution tends to remain in the transverse and ascending colon. If he or she lies on the left side, the solution flows along the ascending colon, down the transverse, and into the sigmoid, causing a sense of urgency to void.) Some women with vaginal, cervical, or uterine tumors take at least one of their daily doses vaginally in a water suspension prepared as above. Those interested in taking shark cartilage via retention enema, might wish to investigate an effective system for administering such enemas developed by Real-Life Products. For further information, call 800–547–6649.

The most dramatic shark cartilage therapy results have been seen with those who were considered "goners," patients for whom all conventional therapies had failed. The patients in the Cuban trial (see pages 95–98), for instance, had been given only months to live. Prior to the trial, each had been treated unsuccessfully with conventional therapies.

In no case has shark cartilage been recommended as an alternative to conventional therapy. Rather, it has been taken in conjunction with conventional therapy, or when all other therapies have failed. Personally, I feel very strongly that cancer patients should not replace conventional therapy with shark cartilage. I do believe that the cartilage can and probably should be used in addition to conventional therapies, in which case, the dosage of shark cartilage should remain constant until the tumors are gone.

One physician who has been monitoring her patients' use of shark cartilage in conjunction with conventional therapy is Barbara Seligman, M.D., director of medical oncology at Flushing Hospital in Queens, New York. "I see no drawbacks to using shark cartilage along with chemotherapy," says Dr. Seligman, who has also used shark cartilage as the sole treatment with some cancer patients. She began working with shark cartilage because she was impressed with audio tapes prepared by me and given to her by a patient. "I have strong positive feelings about the therapeutic value of shark cartilage," she says. "The premise and theory are absolutely correct. Just consider that pharmaceutical companies are now looking for exactly the kind of antiangiogenic agents proposed by Dr. Lane."

Dr. Seligman has reported improvement in patients with whom she has worked, noting in particular one woman whose tumor shrunk and whose psoriasis cleared. She also says she cannot at this time offer more statistics to back up her belief in shark cartilage because so few of her patients have stuck with the therapy. Many patients have found the taste and smell of the powdered shark cartilage objectionable. (When large doses are called for, the tablet form is not practical.) Luckily, a relatively new high-quality shark cartilage product that is practically tasteless and odorless is now available. This product, which is being used in one of the FDA-approved trials, is almost 45 percent protein.

Dr. Seligman administers 80 to 100 grams of powdered shark cartilage to patients with metastatic disease. For those who have had surgery for breast cancer, Dr. Seligman advises using a daily maintenance dose of 10 to 15 grams of shark cartilage in tablet form. She believes this will prevent any remaining tumor cells from developing the blood network needed for their growth.

Of course, finding an "orthodox" medical practitioner who will work with shark cartilage may not be easy. Many physicians are simply not familiar with the work that has been done and is currently being done. Ultimately, however, your health is your responsibility. You can accomplish the goals you desire by having the appropriate information, formulating a plan of action, and being persistent. (See Chapter 10, "Talking To Your Doctor.") Knowing that shark cartilage is completely nontoxic is important to your arsenal of information.

POSSIBLE SIDE EFFECTS

During the Cuban trials, x-ray images of the intestines were taken before and after administration of the cartilage. "No damage can be said to have been found," says Dr. Menendez. In all of the trials, the product has generally been well-tolerated by the patients, who ranged in age from the teens to the eighties. Oral administration appears to cause no irritation, bleeding, or damage to the walls of the stomach or intestine. The lack of side effects was observed regardless of the dosage, but higher doses sometimes caused gas.

Recently, a new form of shark cartilage has been developed in Australia using a unique organic process (see page 194). This product, in which the protein is highly concentrated, does not seem to cause gastric disturbances and has no unpleasant odor. For some, it may be difficult to get around the mild fishlike taste of the protein material. However, because this product is highly concentrated, the product can be taken in smaller doses than other brands. This quality shark cartilage, which is distributed by a Woodcliff Lake, New Jersey laboratory, is one of the two products being used in the current FDA-approved trials.

CANCERS THAT RESPOND TO SHARK CARTILAGE

I am frequently asked what kinds of cancers are expected to respond to shark cartilage. The cartilage should, theoretically, be most effective against fast-growing, highly vascularized tumors, such as those of the breast, cervix, central nervous system, and liver. Shark cartilage therapy has been shown to be highly effective on advanced prostate tumors, and it usually dramatically lowers PSA number (a solid tumor marker) within twelve to sixteen weeks. We have also found that shark cartilage works best on solid tumors; 50 percent of such tumors consist of blood vessels and interstitial space (space between

Exercising Your Options

When illness or adversity strike, some turn for succor to others. Some turn inward, to themselves. Still others turn to God. For Sister Michelle Teff, of the Association of Consecrated Virgins, the choice was clear-cut. She has devoted her life to the love of God and to caring for His people. For her, caring has been more than devotion to people's spiritual needs; as a fully trained chiropractor, she has also devoted herself to people's physical needs. And as a chiropractor, she is well aware of options in alternative medicine.

When Sister Michelle's surgeon found a 3cm-x-2cm malignant tumor in her breast, he insisted that she have a radical mastectomy as soon as possible, warning that without it the breast cancer would likely spread throughout her body within one month. She immediately checked herself out of the hospital.

Sister Michelle was well aware of the consequences of surgery. "There are many, many who have surgery and whose cancer cells spread via their blood." And she did not see radiation and/or chemotherapy as viable alternatives either. She believed that many patients suffer more from these toxic treatments than from the illness itself. Sister Michelle simply believed there had to be a better way to deal with her illness, "I decided to take my chances and put my faith in God."

Sister Michelle has always felt that there is much in nature to heal and sustain us. "We've come so far, we've lost sight of nature. We rely on pharmaceuticals, on artificial cures, instead of turning to nature, to those things that are in harmony with our bodies."

In the hour of her adversity, Sister turned to Dr. Edward Ellis of Greenwich, Connecticut, a naturopathic physician with whom she was personally acquainted and for whom she held a deep respect. "When at Dr. Ellis' I would see cancer patients, gravely ill people who had to be helped to walk out of the office. As time *passed, I would see the same people improving, getting stronger. It was like watching a miracle unfold before your eyes." Sister learned that these people were using shark cartilage.*

On the basis of Dr. Ellis' suggestions, Sister Michelle decided to begin a daily regimen of shark cartilage and botanicals. Within four months of taking BeneFin shark cartilage as well as a number of botanicals, her tumor—one that was considered quite large— had begun to shrink. Sister Michelle is thankful that she didn't pursue traditional therapies before using shark cartilage. "I think," she says, "my body would have been too depressed to respond to the cartilage if I had done that."

When asked if she experienced any negative side effects from the cartilage, Sister replied, "I was really tired, exhausted actually, but I believe that was because my body was trying to heal itself and not due to the cartilage. I also had stomach cramps and felt nauseated. Again, I think those were the results of the body trying to get rid of toxicity. We tend to think of cramping and nausea as negatives, but they are positive signs of the body's elimination of toxic materials." Sister has been taking shark cartilage for nine months. She takes five tablets a day as a maintenance dose and, to date, has been declared 97 percent cancer free.

Although Sister Michelle's parents and siblings were very supportive of her decision, one brother, who is pursuing a career in traditional health care, thought she was taking too great a risk. Some of her friends also thought she was just killing herself because she wasn't approaching her disease with traditional medicine. But Sister Michelle had the courage of her conviction that shark cartilage, a natural product, was the means by which she would get better.

Now she hopes to get the word out and touch as many lives as possible. "If I can do anything to give people options, I will. I want to invite people to another possibility; have the courage to explore all the possibilities. The more options of which we are aware, the more we can exercise our human freedom."

cells). These, then, are the tumors most likely to be affected in a positive way by inhibition of angiogenesis.

In the trials conducted thus far, shark cartilage has worked well against breast and prostate cancer, the number-one cancer killers in women and men respectively. Prostate tumors have been reduced by 15 to 67 percent, PSA has been lowered almost to zero, and quality of life has been improved in nearly 100 percent of the cases. Breast cancer patients have had similar experiences and many are now cancer-free.

Since they started working with patients, doctors have observed positive responses with pancreatic cancer patients taking, in general, 2 grams of shark cartilage per kilogram of body weight daily—providing these patients are still fairly healthy. Normally, unless the cancer is discovered very early, the chances of recovery from pancreatic cancer through conventional therapy are highly limited.

Physicians have often seen responses in liver and renal cancer as well. One of the most rewarding moments for me came during a presentation at the Eighth International Breast Cancer Conference held in Rio de Janeiro, Brazil. A physician told those in attendance about her husband who had been diagnosed with advanced renal cancer and was passing blood and losing weight. Because of a television show I had been on in Brazil, the doctor called me for more information. Within a short time, her husband started to take shark cartilage. Twelve weeks later, he was gaining weight, had stopped passing blood, and appeared to be on his way to recovery.

Although shark cartilage has no effect on AIDS per se, it seems to work on Kaposi's sarcoma, a related skin cancer. An FDA-approved clinical trial of shark cartilage's effect on this condition is currently underway.

With shark cartilage therapy, we have seen a pretty consistent reduction of ovarian tumors. Uterine, cervical, and central nervous system cancers also seem to be among the cancers that respond positively. X-rays have confirmed no regrowth of central nervous system tumors that had been surgically removed. Normally, as stated in the *Mayo Clinic Family Health Disc*, unless the tumor tissue is totally excised during surgery, "recurrence is likely."

OTHER CONDITIONS THAT RESPOND TO SHARK CARTILAGE

Tumors and metastases are not the only conditions for which shark cartilage appears effective. Many people who have been using shark cartilage as a cancer therapy, have also reported a notable improvement in other conditions such as rheumatoid and osteoarthritis, psoriasis, and enteritis.

Remember, it is believed that shark cartilage works against tumors because of its antiangiogenic properties—its ability to halt the development of blood vessels. In addition to cancer, there are actually a host of diseases that have been called "angiogenic." These include the aforementioned conditions, as well as diabetic retinopathy, neovascular glaucoma, and the form of macular degeneration known as "wet." Because these diseases are associated with the development of new blood vessels, it is probable that shark cartilage may be effective in their treatment. Indeed, researchers, physicians, and patients have had successes with psoriasis and arthritis—particularly rheumatoid arthritis.

It has been observed that osteoarthritis pain is alleviated with a daily dose of 1 gram of shark cartilage powder for every 15 pounds of body weight, or one 740- to 750-milligram tablet for each 11 pounds of body weight. Once the pain has been relieved, 1 gram of powder per 40 pounds of body weight appears to be a good daily maintenance dose. If there is no pain relief within thirty days, suspend the treatment. This is a sign that the treatment is not working.

The role of angiogenesis in eye disease has recently been

confirmed by researchers. Working independently, Lloyd Paul
Aiello, M.D., an opthamologist at the Joslin Diabetes Center in
Boston, and opthamologist Anthony Adamis, M.D., at Massachusetts Eye and Ear Infirmary and Children's Hospital in
Boston, have shown that abnormal growth of capillaries
(angiogenesis) leads to the bleeding, tearing, and scarring of
the retina that results in blindness. The researchers were able
to block eye damage in monkeys and mice with injections of
synthetic antibodies. Their studies indicate that the damage
which leads to diabetic retinopathy can be halted with injected
proteins. Dr. Aiello believes that someday oral drugs may be
used to halt the angiogenesis that causes eye damage.

For wet macular degeneration and neovascular glaucoma, 1
gram of powder per 15 pounds of body weight appears to have a
prophylactic effect. This dosage, given daily, seems to stop the
development of small blood vessels before damage is done.

When used to treat enteritis, 1 gram of shark cartilage per
15 pounds of body weight is administered daily. Relief has been
seen in less than 30 days.

In the treatment of psoriasis as well as rheumatoid arthritis,
there has been improvement when 20 to 30 grams (increasing
with weight) of shark cartilage is taken daily for 60 to 90 days.
All the daily doses appear to be most effective when they are
divided into 3 equal parts, with each part taken 30 minutes
before meals.

PROPHYLACTIC POSSIBILITIES

According to angiogenesis theory, it should also be possible
to use shark cartilage prophylactically (as a preventive). The
prophylactic effect is only theoretical; no studies have been
done yet. Trials of prophylactic effects are very costly, requiring
large numbers of subjects who are followed over many years.
Such trials are usually run with government funding, some-

thing I have not enjoyed. I have, however, spoken with many people, particularly women, who have used the cartilage to reduce the chances of metastasis or recurrence of cancer.

One young woman had undergone surgery in 1988 for cancer of the breast and lymph nodes. Although the prognosis following the operation was not good, this young woman read about shark cartilage, questioned me extensively, and decided to use the cartilage. She takes nine capsules (slightly less then 7 grams) per day, and encourages those in similar situations to do likewise. Considering that the odds of developing a recurrence of the cancer within two years are 30 percent, and neither this woman nor those whom she has counseled have experienced that recurrence, it appears that 7 to 8 grams of shark cartilage daily may have prophylactic benefit. Of course, a sound lifestyle including good nutrition and maintenance of ideal body weight must be pursued at the same time.

CAUTIONS AND CONSIDERATIONS

Please be aware that the dosage levels used in the trials are very different from the levels for a dietary supplement described on bottles of shark cartilage products currently being marketed. These dosages are usually based on average calcium or phosphorus supplements. Be aware, too, that the dosage needed to elicit a response will vary with the product used. The amount of active protein being delivered will depend on the purity and the processing method of the product used, many of which contain flavors, sugar, and other dilutants (see Chapter 11). Consider carefully how much active protein is delivered by a product that is 45 percent sugar or 99.27 percent water. Remember, the FDA has not approved generic shark cartilage for clinical trials but rather two specific products that are processed in specific ways. To get FDA approval for clinical trials, the detailed processing methods had to be carefully spelled out.

Giving Life the Green Light

Living with illness is nothing new to Yoriko "Ruth" Bynum. The fifty-nine-year-old resident of Alabama has a long history of liver disease and diabetes. But it wasn't until the summer of 1993 that another illness threatened to take her life.

At that time, Ruth began to experience a persistent cough and shortness of breath. Preliminary tests revealed that she had metastatic lung cancer (bilateral pulmonary metastatic disease). To some, that diagnosis sounds like a death sentence. Those people go home, put their affairs in order, and simply wait. Not Ruth. Not her family.

Ruth's daughter Dona Stracener is a registered nurse with many years of experience in pediatric intensive care. Both she and her sister Annette Jones understood the need for highly trained medical professionals, advanced technology, and an awareness of recent medical developments. So they sought the services of Michael W. Meshad, M.D., a well-known oncologist.

Dr. Meshad, who felt Ruth's prognosis was "extremely poor," recommended against chemotherapeutic intervention due to its toxicity and the disastrous effect it would have on Ruth's liver condition. At this time, Ruth's cancer was causing her marked breathing difficulties, a nonproductive cough, and swelling of the feet. Increasing distention and tightness in her abdomen were causing her discomfort. She was receiving oxygen through a nasal tube to help her breathe, Loratab to suppress her cough and relieve her pain, and Librax, an antianxiety drug, to help her rest at night.

Still, drawing upon inner strength and determination, Ruth and her family did not despair. They turned, instead, to the renowned M.D. Anderson Cancer Clinic in Houston, Texas. Here, the disease was considered "fairly extensive" in degree. A colonoscopy and upper endoscopy were performed, but a primary source of the cancer was not identified. An ultrasound of the abdomen did reveal a possible mass in the head of the pancreas.

The diagnosis of bilateral lung cancer was confirmed by x-rays, a CAT scan, and a lung biopsy. Like Dr. Meshad, the physician at the center recommended against chemotherapy. Ruth's prognosis was not good: the cancer was aggressive and her history of liver disease made the use of chemotherapy dangerous. During her stay at the medical center, Ruth received oxygen for increasing difficulty in breathing, and it was necessary for her to use a wheelchair.

Ruth's return to Alabama was somber. Hope seemed to be dimming. Dr. Meshad sensed the family's despair and recognized how little conventional medicine could do for his patient. He, therefore, suggested that the family consider the unconventional and nontoxic shark cartilage treatments. Family members read **Sharks Don't Get Cancer** *and began to hope again.*

Shark cartilage treatments for Ruth were administered by the family. She was given approximately 20 grams (3 rounded teaspoons) of shark cartilage powder mixed with water, four times a day via rectal retention enemas. (This dosage was based on 1 gram of powder per two pounds of her body weight.) To maintain a fairly high level of active protein in Ruth's bloodstream, doses were given to her in the early morning, mid-morning, mid-afternoon, and at bedtime.

In the second week of the treatments, Ruth noticed that the arthritic pain she had been experiencing in the small finger of the her left hand was completely gone. By the fourth week, Ruth's once constant, nonproductive cough, became intermittant and productive. She was able to get around with only minimal assistance and needed less oxygen than she had previously required. Each day, improvement was noted.

During Ruth's monthly examination on October 22, 1993, Dr. Meshad was amazed to find that she no longer exhibited difficulty in breathing and was fully ambulatory. The oxygen and prescribed medications were eliminated along with the wheelchair. Ruth's physical exam showed her lungs to be clear, and a chest x-ray revealed nearly complete resolution of her pulmonary metastatic disease. Subsequent x-rays taken on January 11, 1994, document nearly complete remission. The doctor's records for that date read:

- *Lung fields show near complete resolution of the bilateral extensive pulmonary metastatic disease originally diagnosed in August with marked decrease in Oct. and further decrease today such that they are barely visible.*
- *IMPRESSION: DRAMATIC RESOLUTION OF BILATERAL METASTATIC ADENOCARCINOMA. [Capital letters are the doctor's.]*

By April of 1994, the doctor's notations indicate that there is an area in Ruth's left lung that may be "vascular shadow or residual tumor. The remainder of her lesions have melted away."

With her strength and spirit so fully restored, Ruth was able to take a long-planned trip to her birthplace—Japan. She continues to take shark cartilage once a day on a prophylactic basis so that her plans for the future will not "melt away" but will come to fruition.

One of these products is a new highly active shark cartilage product. Recently introduced on the market, this product is unique in that it is approximately 42 percent highly effective protein. All indications are that the dosage with this product can be reduced by 25 to 35 percent over shark cartilage that averages 31 to 35 percent protein. The reduced dosage levels will give equal responses with a reduction in the amount needed as well as in the cost. Studies now underway will suggest whether the dosage can be reduced even further based on the rapid absorption rates as well as the higher active protein content. Another benefit of this product is that it is almost tasteless and odorless.

There are times when people do not want to inhibit angiogenesis. Shark cartilage should, therefore, not be used by those who are pregnant or attempting to become pregnant, or by those who have circulatory problems that require the formation of collateral blood vessels, such as those required after blockage of coronary vessels. The cartilage should not be used for thirty days before or after major surgery—a period when angiogenesis plays a vital role in healing the body. It is, however, probably all right to use shark cartilage before a biopsy specimen is taken. In each case, individuals must consider the risk of dying from cancer as opposed to other health risks. Patients should discuss the possibilities with their doctors.

Remember, shark cartilage is not a miracle elixir. Patients hear about dramatic results and often anticipate an immediate improvement in their own conditions. After a week or two, they become disappointed and impatiently change the treatment. *I cannot stress enough the need for patience.* Shark cartilage excites a natural or biological response, a slower response than that of chemotherapy or radiation.

Advanced cancer patients can expect to wait six to eight weeks for a response. First, there will be an improvement in quality of life (i.e. improved stamina), then patients can expect pain reduction, and only later, tumor changes. Patients must be sure that they are taking a sufficiently high dose; the three to six daily capsules taken by some who are receiving incorrect information falls far short of the dosage that has been shown necessary.

Unfortunately, investigators are finding that only about 20 percent of those who start on shark cartilage therapy stay with it for the twenty weeks needed to achieve results. Some people give it up because they feel the shark cartilage has too unpleasant a taste and odor. For many, the high cost of the therapy is a factor. Since there is no insurance coverage for such therapy or for food supplements, the out-of-pocket expense is significant. Shark cartilage is, however, far less expensive a therapy than radiation, chemotherapy, or surgery. Shark cartilage therapy costs between

$4,000 and $7,000 for the first twenty weeks depending on body weight, and about $100 per month for preventive use. Compare this to the cost of surgery (approximately $75,000), or to a series of radiation treatments (approximately $50,000), or chemotherapy treatments (approximately $60,000). Rapidly escalating health-care costs dramatically demonstrate the need for inexpensive therapies such as shark cartilage.

Remember, too, that shark cartilage should not be viewed as a substitute for conventional therapy; instead, it may be considered as an adjunct to conventional treatments. As a matter of fact, Bruce Zetter, M.D., professor of surgery at Children's Hospital, Harvard Medical School, believes that chemotherapy can be used to attack a tumor directly while antiangiogenic therapies can be used to attack it indirectly. Dr. Zetter points out that the body will not build up resistance to antiangiogenic therapies as it can with other treatment modalities. This is a major point because with chemo and radiation therapy, resistance builds quickly and the beneficial effects disappear. Other physicians, such as Dr. Robert Atkins, host of the "Dr. Atkins Show" on New York's WOR radio, feel strongly that chemotherapy impedes the effect of shark cartilage. He, in fact, opposes the use of any chemotherapy on the grounds that it destroys the immune system, the body's natural and first line of defense.

We are simply not certain at this time whether shark cartilage can interfere with other treatments or vice versa. There is, though, no evidence to suggest the cartilage might interfere. Many physicians say they have no real reason for not recognizing the simultaneous administration of shark cartilage and conventional therapies, and scores of people are now using shark cartilage in conjunction with conventional therapies. During clinical trials, however, shark cartilage therapy must not be used with other therapies. Results must be attributable only to the substance being tested. In practice, if a patient uses a combination of therapies and gets results, that's great. It doesn't matter who or what gets the credit.

THE DIGESTION ISSUE

Central to the issue of shark cartilage's efficacy as an orally administered tumor-inhibitor is the question of whether it can be absorbed and get to work in the bloodstream before being digested. During digestion, nutrients are broken down to simpler chemical compounds. A protein, a large or "macro" molecule that consists of long sequences of amino acids, is broken down from polypeptide to proteose to peptone (or peptide) to amino acid. As you may recall, the evidence indicates that the active component of cartilage is a whole protein (or proteins) and not that protein's constituent amino acids.

Many medical people are skeptical about the efficacy of shark cartilage because they believe that the proteins responsible for antiangiogenesis will be digested—broken down to their constituent amino acids, which are not antiangiogenic—before they can have a therapeutic effect. Current research in the digestion and assimilation of proteins indicates that this fear is *not* well grounded. In fact, there is a therapeutic system in use today that actually uses an orally ingested protein to combat disease. Oral tolerization occurs when foreign proteins enter the body through the digestive system and suppress immune responses rather than trigger them. Oral tolerization was first used as a therapy for humans suffering from multiple sclerosis who were fed myelin, a brain substance. Researchers have now fed the protein collagen to arthritis patients with good success (see pages 137–138).

Consider, too, that in *Physiology of the Gastrointestinal Tract*, David Alpers, M.D., points to numerous cases in which it is known that small peptides cross the intestine and enter the circulation. He contends that there is no doubt of the widespread nature of this phenomenon.

We know that the digestibility of proteins differs, but we do not know all of the factors that affect digestion and, therefore, determine the differences. "Traditionally, amino acids are always regarded as the fundamental 'currency' of protein metabolism," writes biochemist Dr. Michael Gardner of the University of Edinburgh Medical School. It is commonly believed that it is predominantly free amino acids that enter the portal circulation (the route by which blood passes through veins that break into a capillary network) before returning to the heart.

Consider, however, that in one experiment, removal of 70 percent of the small intestine of rats did *not* affect protein digestion. As Dr. Gardner puts it, ". . . there is now a substantial body of evidence, albeit not widely known, that significant quantities of larger molecules, including peptides and even intact proteins, can cross the intestine." He says that even though the intestinal epithelium is often regarded as an absolute barrier that prevents macromolecules from entering the systemic circulation, there is "abundant evidence" that a variety of macromolecules and even particulate matter cross the intestine. Dr. Gardner is one of many who believes that the apparent lack of peptides in portal blood may be the result of technical problems in detecting the peptides. He feels that there are problems with the process involved in marking a protein in order to track that protein during a biological process such as digestion.

Dr. Gardner points out that many researchers today do acknowledge that some intact protein may be absorbed in peripheral tissues where it might be biologically active. Brian Blackadar, M.D., a professor of nutritional sciences in a Canadian university, believes that components of shark cartilage may also enter the bloodstream and be transported to a cancer site. In other words, an orally ingested protein might exert a biological effect on a tumor outside the gastrointestinal tract.

According to Dr. Gardner, there are some researchers who believe that absorption of intact proteins actually proceeds on a rather large scale. He points to scientist Dr. W. Hemmings who has repeatedly said that large amounts of undegraded or partly degraded protein do cross the intestine. One example of absorption of a biologically active protein is provided by botulism: the toxin is so potent that absorption of a very minute quantity is lethal.

Although digestion is an efficient process that delivers most of the protein products to the portal vein (the vein that passes blood into the liver from the digestive system) in the form of free amino acids, exceptions have been found. Investigators have demonstrated that a protein extracted from soybeans (the Bowman Birk protease inhibitor or BBI) becomes widely distributed in the tissue of mice following oral feeding through a stomach tube. Using radioactive techniques, researchers at the University of Pennsylvania School of Medicine showed BBI was present in the mice's serum, esophagus, stomach and intestine, liver, and lungs. The highest levels of radioactivity were seen in the contents obtained from the stomach, small bowel, and colon.

The total amount of the labeled material found in the blood was 4.7 to 5.9 percent. Researchers found that BBI is transported across the small intestinal mucosa, is absorbed, and becomes widely distributed. Figure 9.1 shows the distribution of BBI three hours after administration. It was also found that the labeled BBI obtained from animal tissues is the same size as that originally administered to the animals. Significantly, researchers concluded, "The BBI present in the colon could be delivered via the bloodstream or be directly absorbed from the intestinal lumen by the colonic epithelium."

The Bowman Birk experiments, which were supported by NIH grants, are indicative of new digestion research being conducted in living animals. Much of the information regarding the overall processes of digestion and absorption of carbohydrates and protein had been obtained *in vitro*—in an environment created outside the living body. Such studies provide very useful information, but they may not completely reveal the events that occur within the living body. According to Dr. Alpers, a great deal of work must be done before the *in vivo* utilization of foodstuffs is really understood.

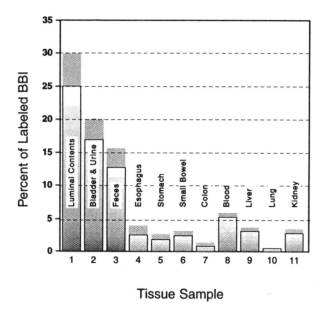

Figure 9.1. Distribution of Bowman Birk Protease Inhibitor (BBI).
BBI, a protein derived from soybeans, becomes widely distributed in tissues
of mice following oral feeding through a stomach tube. The results presented
above show the percentage of the total protein found.

Researchers in the Combined Program in Pediatric Gastroenterology and Nutrition at Massachusetts General Hospital
and the Children's Hospital affiliated with Harvard Medical
School, report that some dietary proteins (the proteins we eat)
are absorbed and serve as antigens (substances foreign to the
body). The intestine actually surveys antigens by allowing
small quantities to cross the intestinal epithelium (covering)
and interact with the mucosal and immune system. In other
words, one of the ways in which the body recognizes materials
that require activation of the immune system is by sampling. In
order to get the samples, the body permits substances—some
of which are certain to be proteins that are three-quarters of the
dry weight of most cell matter—to enter the vascular system.

The researchers report that specialized epithelial cells have characteristics that enable them to transport intact antigens. They have, for instance, shown that when children who are allergic to milk are "challenged with milk," the protein macromolecules enter their circulation.

Furthermore, there are some essential macromolecules that are taken up by the intestinal epithelium directly from the lumen of the bowel. Certain transepithelial mechanisms facilitate the uptake of such proteins as growth factors and immunoglobulins. Some growth factors must be taken up by the intestine and transported into the circulation. This is often achieved by the growth factors' binding to specific receptors that can shuttle them across the intestine without their being broken into simpler compounds. In short, growth factors—proteins—enter the circulation *without being digested*. After all, the development of the small intestine depends on several growth factors, some of which are delivered from the circulation, some of which enter the intestinal lining directly from the gastrointestinal tract.

Dr. Alpers notes that some proteins are resistant to fragmentation by addition of water (proteolysis) and almost completely escape digestion in the alimentary tract. The best documented of these is intrinsic factor, which is produced in the stomach and combines with vitamin B_{12} to form an antianemic principle. Dr. Alpers further states that "normal intestinal transit may not permit the time necessary for hydrolysis to amino acids and small peptides to occur for all proteins." It is most interesting to note that certain dipeptides which contain residues of an amino acid that is a major constituent of collagen, a protein abundant in cartilage, are absorbed intact.

Dr. Gardner points out that people with congenital problems involving the intestinal transport of amino acids can absorb those acids well when they are presented as dipeptides. He writes, "It is now certain that some small peptides, some macromolecules including proteins and some inert particles *can* and do cross the healthy small intestine *in vivo* in intact form."

(The emphasis is his.) It is interesting to note that macromolecules adhere to the surface of immature cells more readily than to mature cells. If, therefore, the active principle in shark cartilage is a macromolecule, it might very well adhere more to rapidly developing tumor cells. Any effect the macromolecule might have on cells would be enhanced in tumor cells.

I discussed the body's ability to absorb "whole proteins" the size of the active components in shark cartilage during a visit to the National Institutes of Health in 1991. Dr. Robert Gallo clearly stated, to my pleasant surprise, that particles up to 45,000 daltons (a dalton is $\frac{1}{12}$ the mass of a carbon-12 atom) can be absorbed by the digestive system of a cancer patient. It has been noted that the active proteins in shark cartilage probably do not exceed 15,000 daltons and can definitely be absorbed as an undigested whole. Yet people concerned with theories continue to criticize and challenge my work.

There are also physicians who are concerned about the possibility of hypercalcemia (an abnormally high concentration of calcium in the blood) in patients who take shark cartilage. The calcium content in whole shark cartilage is high, and patients use a lot of it. I have discussed the problem with many physicians who have treated hundreds of cancer patients. Many doctors say hypercalcemia is common with advanced cancer and shark cartilage therapy, but none of them, to my knowledge, has seen negative effects as a result of the high calcium level. If conventional therapies have failed a terminal cancer patient, a degree of hypercalcemia may be an acceptable risk. Only the patient and his or her doctor can or should decide, but they should keep open minds.

IN CONCLUSION

Preliminary findings indicate that malignant as well as benign tumors shrink as a result of the administration of shark cartilage, and that quality of life is almost always improved. There is also a sizable body of evidence indicating that shark cartilage alleviates the pain and inflammation associated with arthritis. Theoretically, the cartilage should work against other angiogenesis-dependant diseases such as diabetic retinopathy, wet macular degeneration, and psoriasis. The results will vary depending on how advanced the disease is, on concurrent treatments, and on the amount and brand of material being used. The route of administration does not, however, appear to be a factor.

The best news from the trials that have been conducted to date may be that we've administered thousands upon thousands of doses of shark cartilage with no adverse reactions, no toxicity. Lack of toxicity is a significant breakthrough when one considers the debilitating effects of the traditional cancer therapies—radiation, chemotherapy, and surgery. Cancer specialist Charles B. Simone, M.D., is quoted in the October 26, 1993, issue of *Women's World* as saying that shark cartilage is "a totally nontoxic treatment with no side effects and it's getting a response equal to or better than most chemotherapies."

Most chemotherapies—as scores of people know too well— have incredibly debilitating side effects such as extreme fatigue, hair loss, and nausea. These therapies are almost as toxic to the patients as they are to the tumors they destroy—if they destroy them. Indeed, they are called *cytotoxic drugs*—drugs that are toxic to or poison cells.

Because shark cartilage is a nontoxic product, I've taken the stand that we can't hurt anybody. All we can do is help people. I feel this gives us the liberty to move faster, especially with terminal patients, than many scientists would like us to. When faced with 600,000 Americans dying each year (more than the total number of United States soldiers killed in World War II and Vietnam combined), how can we *slowly* study a safe, non-invasive, relatively inexpensive substance that so many are using effectively?

It is, in the final analysis, up to you to make the decisions that affect your well-being. You must weigh the advantages and disadvantages of using shark cartilage, and proceed with caution.

10.

Talking to Your Doctor

It's not what you say, it's how you say it.

It is very important to work with a physician when you are taking shark cartilage. There are two basic reasons. First, it is important to monitor your condition so that changes can be made in your treatment when necessary. Secondly, when enough physicians begin to document the improvements brought about by shark cartilage, it will be more difficult for establishment medical authorities to dismiss the growing body of evidence as anecdotal.

There may be a problem in getting your physician to work with you, but, if you have a serious condition for which you want to try shark cartilage, you are going to have to deal with a physician. If there's one thing I've learned during my years of trying to get shark cartilage tested, it's that the right approach combined with organization and persistence—in that order— are the only tools for opening doors. You might do well to begin by thinking of the cliché with which this chapter opens. Too often, we find ourselves agreeing with those words with a sense of regret when we have spoken in haste. Remember, belligerence and hostility will not get you what you want, and advanced cancer patients have no time for regrets.

Whatever you do, don't let despair kill you before you're dead. Consider the story of Jack V. LaChapelle, a cancer survivor. He recounts, "I was caught between professional opinions. I alone had to make the choice; my life could depend on the decision. . . . The risks were high, a 10% to 25% chance of success. . . . The senior general surgeon at the hospital did not want to operate. . . . I brought out [literature about the operation]; I recounted the internist's recommendation. I pressed him to operate. . ." After weighing all of the facts, Mr. LaChapelle got the operation he wanted and success was his.

Remember, there is a significant difference between positive mental attitude and blind or false hope. If you have a positive attitude, you recognize that you have a life-threatening disease. You recognize, too, that there is always a chance to beat it, but you may not get a second chance. You must, therefore, find out all you can about your particular cancer—all of the statistics, available treatments, qualified doctors. Make a commitment to fighting your disease. But do not wear a blindfold by simply saying, I will get well." Actively go after the medical treatments and other options that might help. And one of the most important steps is to find the physician who is best for you.

ARM YOURSELF WITH KNOWLEDGE

Before discussing the possibilities of shark cartilage therapy with a doctor, there are basically two things that you should do. First, be prepared. It is important to be knowledgeable about shark cartilage before your appointment. And second, use the right approach when discussing this subject with the doctor. Don't simply go to your doctor and tell him or her that you want to use shark cartilage because you heard about it from your cousin Fred. It is crucial for you to know something about the subject. You should be well versed on the principles and the history of this therapy. If you have a good understanding of shark cartilage, you will be in a better position to explain it.

Be familiar with the following important facts:

- *The theory behind shark cartilage's use as an antitumor agent is sound and well established.* In *The New England Journal of Medicine* in 1971, Dr. Judah Folkman of Children's Hospital and Harvard Medical School postulated that tumor development and growth can be arrested by cutting off the tumor's blood supply. Researchers such as Drs. Robert Langer and Anne Lee of the Massachusetts Institute of Technology subsequently proved the efficacy of the theory in laboratory experiments.

- *Shark cartilage is nontoxic.* The Chinese have been eating shark-fin soup for thousands of years with no evidence of harmful side effects. In fact, the rate of certain kinds of cancer is lower among Chinese people than among Westerners. In clinical trials conducted in Panama, Mexico, and Cuba, more than 122 cancer patients used shark cartilage with no side effects except for a few cases of gastric distress. Currently, United States FDA approved clinical trials are being conducted or are about to begin in New Jersey and Michigan under two INDs from the FDA. Again, no adverse side effects are being reported.

- *Shark cartilage appears to be an effective therapeutic agent.* In the Mexican trials conducted in 1991, seven of eight terminal cancer patients experienced significant tumor reduction (five patients showed 100 percent reduction, two had 80 percent reduction, and only one showed no response). Of the terminal patients who used shark cartilage in the Cuban clinical trails conducted in 1992–93, 48 percent experienced significant improvement in their conditions and were alive, well, and active as of the writing of this book.

- *Shark cartilage has been shown to diminish pain and improve quality of life.* Physicians involved in the clinical trials concur that patients using shark cartilage "dramatically improved their quality of life." Use of the shark cartilage notably reduced pain. Improvement of quality of life may be as important in some ways as is tumor reduction.

- *Shark cartilage can be readily purchased at health food stores.* According to government regulations, it is perfectly legal to buy and take shark cartilage as a food supplement.

Familiarizing yourself with these important facts will help a doctor understand why you want to use shark cartilage as a cancer therapy.

SEARCHING FOR A DOCTOR

You are now ready to look for a physician who will work with you. You should certainly consider the following criteria when selecting a doctor:

- The doctor should be licensed to practice medicine in your state.
- The doctor should have graduated from an accredited institution. (Be aware, however, that the quality of the doctor's education is not the only factor that determines how good he or she is.)
- The doctor should be willing to talk to you in a way you understand.
- The doctor's bedside manner should be acceptable to you. Unfortunately, there are many excellent doctors who lack bedside manner, but feeling comfortable with the doctor may not be important to you. If you are willing to put up

with this type of doctor, that's fine. If, however, you believe that a physician with empathy will help take the strain out of a pressured situation, don't be afraid to go with your instinct.

- Understand the costs involved, and know how much your insurance will cover for the doctor's services.

Upon visiting the physician's office for the first time, you may find it helpful to consider the following:

- Based upon your previous experience, was the examination thorough?
- Is the office clean and well equipped?
- Was everything—diagnoses, test results, treatment options—expressed clearly?
- If the physician recommends further diagnostic tests, ask why they are necessary and if there are any risks involved. Be sure to find out if insurance covers their cost and where the testing will be done.

If the doctor does recommend further diagnostic tests, find out if the physician is affiliated with the lab doing the testing. Unfortunately, some physicians share in the profits of diagnostic labs and may, therefore, recommend testing that is not necessary. Some states have made this practice illegal.

Use the Right Approach

Once you have made a preliminary choice of a doctor, it is time to discuss the possibility of using shark cartilage. Remember, the physician is probably busy. If you plan on having a lengthy conversation, you may be best served by getting an appointment at the end of office hours when the doctor is less likely to be rushed.

Since you may well be in a less-than-calm state during the appointment, you should prepare a list of the points and questions you want to discuss with the doctor. This way, you won't forget anything. And because your emotional reactions may prevent you from truly hearing everything the doctor says, it's a good idea to have someone—a close friend or family member—accompany you to the appointment.

Your approach should be based on the type of reaction you get from your doctor. Your first question should be, "Doctor, do you believe in using alternative therapies?" You will probably get one of three responses:

1. "I do not advocate them at all."
2. "I cannot give you an opinion because I do not have enough information on such therapies."
3. "It depends on what the therapy is and how you feel about it."

Obviously, if your doctor is willing to work with you, together you can begin to outline a treatment plan using shark cartilage. Discover what he or she already knows about this therapy, and share all of the knowledge you have. Provide him or her with available literature. Referring the physician to Chapter 9, "Administration of Shark Cartilage," also may prove to be extremely helpful.

If your doctor doesn't have an immediate objection but feels he or she can't commit to working with an alternative therapy because of a lack of information, by all means share your knowledge. Suggest that he or she read either of my books. Make sure that you pinpoint a time at which the doctor will respond to your request. And don't be put off. If your doctor says he or she will get back to you in a week, and a week becomes two, and two become three, consider finding another doctor who shows more interest.

If your doctor voices a strong negative reaction when asked about alternative therapies, you will have to work to convince him or her of the possible benefits of shark cartilage therapy. Begin by mentioning that you have been reading about the use of shark cartilage as a possible alternative treatment. Inform the doctor that shark cartilage has been found to be nontoxic and has shown great promise in a number of studies. Tell the doctor you would very much appreciate it if he or she would work with and monitor you while you take it.

If your physician's response is negative, chances are it is because he or she doesn't know enough about shark cartilage. If this seems to be the case, share what you know. Summarize the most important facts about shark cartilage (outlined beginning on page 169), and ask if the doctor would be open to reading some of the books or articles on the subject. If the doctor seems to be interested, be sure to supply all pertinent information immediately (see the Bibliography beginning on page 217).

However, if your doctor is familiar with shark cartilage therapy and still has reservations, chances are he or she has strong feelings against the therapy itself. The physician may pose the argument that the proteins responsible for antiangiogenesis will be digested before they can be effective in stopping the growth and development of tumors. Remind the doctor that the digestion of protein is not a totally efficient process. Scientific literature is full of reports of protein fragments and intact proteins from the intestine found in the systemic circulation. (A discussion of proteins and digestion appears on pages 158–163.) Active components of shark cartilage may also escape the digestive process and arrive at a tumor via the bloodstream.

Your physician may be against the treatment simply because it is unproven. Point out that *unproven* doesn't mean *disproven* (see page 32). An unproven therapy may soon be proven effective. There is a world of difference in the meaning of these two words.

You might also point out that in November 1985, *Scientific American* reported that of more than 200,000 people receiving chemotherapy, only a small percentage were being cured. Ask your doctor about the statistics on the survival rate, quality of life, side effects, and pain involved in the therapy options he advocates for you.

Keep in mind that there are two general ways of looking at how effective a treatment is. One is a statistical analysis called a *response rate*. In other words, what percentage of patients get a response? (A response being either shrinkage of a tumor or halting of tumor growth.) Many treatments provide an excellent *initial* response. They shock the tumor and stop its growth, but only temporarily. Tumor tissue often adapts to the treatment and begins to grow again. The effectiveness of the drug frequently decreases as the person builds a tolerance to it or the tumor adapts. In other words, total survival time is not increased.

The second way of looking at the effectiveness of a treatment is to consider the overall survival rate. Does the treatment increase the life expectancy? Shark cartilage has been getting a response rate anywhere from 40 percent in lung cancer patients to 90 percent in those with brain cancer, depending on the size of the tumor and the condition of the patient. Because shark cartilage theoretically acts as an antiangiogenic agent, no resistance to the cartilage will develop. Therefore, the survival rate of those using shark cartilage therapy should exceed that for conventional therapies. To date, about 48 percent of the patients who were involved in the Cuban study are living completely normal lives— not just surviving—more than three and a half years after the trial. All of the physicians who have participated in clinical trials are overwhelmingly impressed by the improvement in each patient's quality of life.

Be aware shark cartilage therapy involves no pain or adverse side effects. Discuss with your doctor the possibility of using shark cartilage as an adjunctive therapy— one used in conjunction with other therapies—as well as an alternative therapy.

If it appears that your physician is still set against your using shark cartilage, ask on what his or her specific objection is based. If the objection is due to assumptions or second-hand information, ask the doctor if he or she believes that a patient is entitled to make an informed choice based on all of the available information. The concept of informed choice is becoming more and more prevalent in the practice of medicine. There is even a proposed Healthcare Rights Amendment to the Constitution that calls for a legal guarantee of "the right to and freedom of choice in self-determination in healthcare." If your doctor does not agree that your health is, ultimately, your own responsibility, you should certainly consider looking for another physician to work with you. Remember, there are many highly qualified physicians who may be somewhat more open-minded, more flexible.

You might consider calling Physician Data Query (PDQ) for help in contacting such physicians. Richard Bloch, a cancer survivor, helped organize the PDQ. Cancer patients and their families can call 800–4–CANCER and request a free printout about every type and stage of cancer. Descriptions of ongoing clinical trials are also available. Through this organization, people can get referrals for a second opinion, as well as information about multidisciplinary second-opinion panels. Members of these panels are cancer experts who will suggest the best treatment available to you after reviewing your files. The services of some of these panels are available free of charge. Many of these services, however, are tied to conventional approaches, and may have little knowledge of alternative therapies such as shark cartilage.

As a matter of fact, even if your physician agrees to work with you while you take shark cartilage, it is still wise to get a second opinion. Be aware that there are people who will take advantage of your desperation. And one way to protect yourself is by getting more than one opinion.

Referrals

If you are now seeking a second opinion, consider focusing on those who practice alternative or holistic medicine. An informative guide, *Options and Health Care*, outlines how to choose a doctor who practices alternative medicine. This publication may be ordered by contacting:

People's Medical Society
462 Walnut Street
Allentown, PA 19102
(610) 770–1670

As Frank Wiewel of People Against Cancer puts it, "Trying to bend an orthodox practitioner around the corner will be tough. On the other hand, any doctor willing to do colonic or chelation therapy should be open to shark cartilage."

People Against Cancer is one organization that has rigid acceptance criteria for the doctors they refer. In order for a doctor to get on this organization's list of referrals, he or she must have evidence—"not necessarily proof, but at least evidence"—to support the claims of his or her treatment. The doctor must present well-organized data that shows a number of patients have benefited from the treatment. Then the evidence is sent for further evaluation to an international physicians' network comprised of doctors who are helping people with cancer in innovative ways. According to Mr. Wiewel, "It makes no difference to me what the physician's claim is. It's just that I know patients can be duped into spending lots of money on worthless treatments. There's always someone ready to take your money." For more information on this organization, contact:

People Against Cancer
PO Box 10
Otho, IA 50569–0010
(515) 972–4444

Many other organizations will provide you with referrals to physicians who are open to unconventional treatments. The following groups offer lists or individual referrals at little or no charge:

**American Association of
Naturopathic Physicians
(AANP)**
2366 Eastlake Avenue East
Suite 322
Seattle, WA 98102
(206) 323–7610

**American College for
Advancement in Medicine
(ACAM)**
PO Box 3427
Laguna Hills, CA 96253
(714) 583–7666
(800) 532–3688

Cancer Control Society
2043 North Berendo Street
Los Angeles, CA 90027
(213) 663–7801

**Foundation for the Advance-
ment of Innovative Medicine
(FAIM)**
2 Executive Boulevard
Suite 404
Suffern, NY 10901
(914) 368–9797
*Referrals in New York, New
Jersey, and Connecticut only.*

**Great Lakes Association of
Clinical Medicine (GLACM)**
1407-B North Wells Street
Chicago, IL 60610
(800) 286–6013

Holistic Health Directory
New Age Journal
42 Pleasant Street
Watertown, MA 02172
(617) 926–0200
(800) 783–7006

**International Association of
Cancer Victors and Friends**
3995 Lynfield Court
College Park, GA 30349–1425
(310) 822–5032

**International Holistic Center
(IHC)**
1042 Willow Creek Road
A111–151
Prescott, AZ 86301
(602) 771–1742

**Nutrition for Optimal Health
Association (NOHA)**
PO Box 380
Winnetka, IL 60093
(708) 786–5326

**Patient Advocates for
Advanced Cancer Treat-
ments, Inc. (PAACT)**
1143 Parmelee N.W.
Grand Rapids, MI 49504
(616) 453–1477

**Planetree Health
Resource Center**
2034 Filmore Street - 2nd Floor
San Francisco, CA 94115
(415) 923–3680

**Rheumatoid Disease
Foundation (RDF)**
5106 Old Harding Road
Franklin, TN 37064
(615) 646–1030

**Price Pottenger Nutrition
Foundation (PPNF)**
PO Box 2614
La Mesa, CA 91943–2614
(619) 574–7763
(800) 366–3748

For the names of physicians currently working with patients who are using shark cartilage, call Information Services at 800–742–7534. The service has a list of at least seventy-five physicians throughout the country who use shark cartilage therapy. Someone on staff will refer you to a physician located in your area.

Try to get the names of several physicians so that you may choose one who most closely matches your needs. Once you have names, you might follow the advice of Jane Heimlich in her book *What Your Doctor Won't Tell You*. Ms. Heimlich advises that before making an appointment, first call doctors' offices and speak with the office manager or secretary. Explain that you are interested in becoming a patient and ask a few basic questions, such as what medical school(s) the doctor attended, how long the doctor has been in practice, what treatments he or she uses, and what the fees are.

Frank Wiewel concurs with this advice: "There are innovative doctors with open minds. Sample ten doctors. Talk to them. Walk through the process of your treatment. Listen to the caveats and cautions."

WARNING

It is important to know that there are unscrupulous physicians who capitalize on other people's tragedies. They may have all the proper accreditation, yet they are more interested in your money than in your health. If a physician is making unrealistic promises, be skeptical. If a physician does not accept any insurance, be suspicious. If the prices seem extremely high, be leery, particularly if others provide the same service at a lesser fee.

Ask to speak to a doctor's other patients. Be cautious if he or she refuses to give you names. And be suspicious if the patients to whom you are referred have just begun seeing the doctor. Be sure to talk to patients who have been seeing the doctor for six months to a year.

You may also wish to consider The American Cancer Society's warning that physicians whose record keeping is weak to nonexistent may be suspect. The society also advises against believing those who claim the treatment is secret or secretly prepared. According to the book *Everyone's Guide to Cancer Therapy*, "New scientific therapies are always made available through meetings, talks and publicity to the entire community of scientists and researchers. The worth of the treatment can be confirmed only when the results of research can be reproduced by others."

THOSE WHO BITE BACK

Perhaps more than any people on Earth, cancer patients and their families need to become educated consumers. Those who have done their homework well have found responsible, capable, caring physicians who will work with shark cartilage. The stories of these indomitable people and of the physicians who stand with them never fail to inspire me.

In Reno, Nevada, an interview with internist Douglas Brody, M.D., appeared in the *Reno Gazette-Journal* on October 17, 1993. Although Dr. Brody's experience with shark cartilage was not extensive, he felt it was "effective." The internist reported that his cancer patients do better when he combines shark cartilage with traditional therapies. Dr. Brody has been treating thirty to forty patients in this way and says that 60 percent of them have shown improvement. Although these patients have not been cured, their appetites have improved, they've lost some symptoms, and there has been some reduction in tumor size.

In the same article, Dr. James Forsythe, an oncologist and assistant clinical professor of internal medicine at the University of Nevada-Reno School of Medicine, says, "I have always had an interest in alternative medicine and have become more open-minded over the years because so many patients have done better than they should. . . . shark cartilage is a new therapy that I am still learning about. . . . I have not seen any toxic effects from this alternative therapy, and it does seem to be beneficial."

And in New York, one patient who did better than he should have is Jacob Mankita, an eighty-five-year-old Brooklyn resident who had been diagnosed with metastatic gall bladder cancer. The diseased organ was removed and he had been treated with both chemotherapy and radiation. Still, he was given only months to live. His wife, Rachel, saw the *60 Minutes* segment on shark cartilage and heard mention of Dr. Charles Simone, an American physician who had accompanied me to Cuba. She tracked him down in New Jersey, and Jacob began using shark cartilage powder. Within weeks, he was feeling healthier. Within months, he was walking two miles a day and saying, "I feel like I've been newly born." In April 1995, the Mankitas were interviewed by New York's FOX-5 News in a televised segment that showed a hale Jacob singing. Also shown were the small plastic sharks that the Mankitas now display atop their china cabinet.

There is also the case of a retired seventy-seven-year-old projects engineer at Wright-Patterson Air Force Base who was diagnosed with bladder cancer in 1991. At that time, surgeons were able to remove three-quarters of the tumor. He says shark cartilage removed the rest.

A forty-six-year-old Ohio woman was diagnosed with breast cancer in 1990. Subsequently, the cancer spread, and she was pronounced terminal. She heard about shark cartilage, researched it, and decided to try it. Although the tumor is still present, it has not grown, and "I'm still here," she says.

These are but a few of the large number of people who believe that there has to be a better way to treat cancer than with cytotoxic therapies. These are people whose convictions are helping to make a difference.

You can make a difference, too. Start with your own life. Whatever therapy you choose to fight your disease, be an active participant in the selection process. Investigate the alternatives, learn as much as you can about each. For each alternative, be certain to find out the success rate for your particular form of the disease; not all forms of disease respond the same. Don't allow yourself to be pushed into any treatment too quickly. Unless you are facing a real emergency—loss of blood, cessation of breathing, bowel obstruction—you more than likely have time to consider alternatives. And don't be pushed into a treatment of which you are not certain. Take the time to find out whether you can expect short- or long-term improvement, reduced pain, and enhanced well-being. And be especially certain to learn what, if any, contraindications exist. Be aware of each therapy's possible side effects and danger signs.

IN CONCLUSION

It is a sad commentary about our health-care system that patients have to fend for themselves in order to get the best possible medical care. The fact is, in medicine, the old adage becomes, "Let the patient beware," and it is only too true. I can tell you, however, that once you have found a physician who is qualified and with whom you can work, you have taken a big step toward helping your condition.

And don't forget the words of cancer-survivor Richard Bloch:

> "You must never give up; you must believe it *all* applies to you."

11.

In the Marketplace

Consumption is the sole end and purpose of all production; and the interest of the producer ought to be attended to only so far as it may be necessary for promoting that of the consumer.

Adam Smith
18th century economist

We live in a free society where competition in the marketplace is encouraged. In the hands of responsible people, competition can lead to better products, lower prices, and reasonable assurances of availability. In the hands of unscrupulous individuals, competition can produce a glut of inferior products that may be ineffective, if not downright dangerous. To cite examples, all you have to do is read a newspaper: substandard replacement parts found in aircraft, tainted meat sold by fast-food chains, and food manufacturers convicted of knowingly selling contaminated baby food.

Of course, only a very few business people are so unscrupulous. Most are quite honest and some are simply copycats. Rather than spend time, effort, and money to develop a new or better product, they simply copy one that is doing well in the marketplace. From natural fruit drinks to weight-reduction mixes to drugs to computers, copycat products abound.

Imitators' products certainly take part of the market away from the original product, thereby cutting into the developer's profits. More serious than the financial loss, however, is the possibility that if the imitation is of poor quality, the developer's good name may "go down" with it.

As I suspected, shark cartilage's growing popularity has brought with it a spate of imitators. Many of these products have been poorly processed and are contaminated by bacteria. Others contain almost nothing but sugar. The existence of such products can be a death knell for shark cartilage.

COPYCAT PRODUCTS PROLIFERATE

According to the March 1994, issue of the *Vitamin Retailer*, "The highly publicized book *Sharks Don't Get Cancer* brought the health benefits of shark cartilage to the general public." *Health Foods Business* magazine reports that response to the *60 Minutes* broadcast regarding the benefits of shark cartilage "has produced an unprecedented amount of interest in the supplement."

The media attention given to the efficacy of shark cartilage has helped its sales to skyrocket. Indeed, it has become one of the industry's hottest new products. The American public has been intrigued by the promising research, as well as by the availability of the product in convenient form.

The demand has led companies to literally jump in with untested and often ineffective shark cartilage products. When the book *Sharks Don't Get Cancer* first appeared, there was only one shark cartilage product on the market; now there are dozens. One company claims it sells $10 million dollars worth of shark cartilage per year. The previously mentioned article in *Vitamin Retailer* indicates that the marketers of shark cartilage are getting the cartilage from more than ten suppliers. People have been purchasing these products in health food stores and are also getting them in the offices of practitioners. People who buy shark cartilage in stores or from ill-informed practitioners often use the wrong dosage and may be taking an untested or diluted product. Many suppliers are more interested in their margin of profit than in the effectiveness of the product.One doctor I worked with early on treated his cancer patients with a quality shark cartilage; he was amazed and pleased with the positive response. Eventually, in an effort to cut costs, he switched them to a cheaper product. Within a short period, the patients began to display signs of deterioration. Perplexed, the doctor had the new product analyzed and discovered it was 99.27 percent water.

WHAT COPYCAT PRODUCTS MEAN FOR THE CONSUMER

Originally, I prepared pure shark cartilage in my kitchen in relatively small amounts. It took me years to plan, test, and execute the development of a viable and safe product. There were years of research, animal studies, and clinical trials. Eventually, I received a use patent and then conducted my research with one specific product.

But people are marketing new products in just weeks; some of them are even marketing products that masquerade as products I endorse by saying things such as "as seen on *60 Minutes*" or "as reported in *Sharks Don't Get Cancer*." One product from Hong Kong even used my picture in its promotional material—a picture copied from the one in my first book. (Threat of a lawsuit stopped that practice.) Unfortunately, most of these suppliers have little knowledge of correct production techniques, which are intricate and took me years to develop.

Central to the concept of free enterprise is having a variety of products so that the consumer becomes the judge and jury; inferior products with higher costs are driven from the market by high-quality products with reasonable costs. Certainly, the consumer must also beware of products professing to have high quality but being offered at low cost. Although there are a few exceptions—as when someone develops more efficient processing—low cost often indicates cut corners. Something has to give when you cut costs. In short, you don't get something for nothing. Actually, you sometimes get *less* than what you bargained for.

With products such as shark cartilage, ingredients and processing techniques become critically important. Processing and the method of sterilization—particularly the use of heat and chemicals—can alter the bioactivity of the proteins responsible for antiangiogenesis. Then, too, processing is antithetical to the whole concept of natural alternatives. And the addition of ingredients may make it seem as if there's something extra in a product when it actually diminishes the amount of protein available. Remember, it is the presence of active protein in shark cartilage, not just the quantity of protein, that produces the positive effect. Active proteins will be present only if the processing does not denature the protein or deliver it in particle sizes that cannot be absorbed.

The concept of a "good" shark cartilage product is not as obscure as it may seem. The comparative merits of shark cartilage products can be evaluated. Initially, I used a CAM assay procedure to evaluate quality. In this kind of laboratory analysis, chicken embryos are injected with the substance being tested and then analyzed to determine if the substance inhibited vascularization. However, I soon found an even more reliable and accurate assay—the endothelial cell assay. In this more sophisticated assay, the cells that make up the lining of blood vessels (endothelial cells) are exposed to a test substance. If the cells do not reproduce rapidly, new blood vessels do not form and the substance is deemed to be an angiogenesis inhibitor. Although slower and much more costly than the CAM, the endothelial cell assay is more reliable. Others in the field confirmed my findings, but I did not announce this change in procedure to the public. It is amusing to me that so many manufacturers are stressing the CAM assay in discussing their products' reliability. How seriously can you take a product that is touting a test deemed out-of-date by most professionals—a fact the manufacturers would know if they kept up with developments.

Finding a shark cartilage product that is pure is not the only problem consumers face. Users of the product must also be aware of how shark cartilage is processed.

In some cases, manufacturers increase the amount of material in the bottle by adding fillers such as dextrin (sugar). It's easy to lower the price if you're not giving the consumers what they pay for. One product is said to be processed to "concentrate the mucopolysaccharides, remove ash and extraneous material, and yield a purified, soluble, shark cartilage product." According to the company that manufactures the product, its process involves shredding, deodorizing, and drying of the cartilage, but that's not all. The product also undergoes digestion, purification, decolorization, filtration, addition of dextrin, and sterilization. The "digestion" spoken of occurs because an enzyme (protease) is used to break down the product so that it will be more soluble. It is highly possible that the enzymatic breakdown also breaks the active protein into its constituent amino acids, which have no antiangiogenic effect.

In any event, an educated consumer (even I can be a copycat) would no doubt think that these products undergo a lot of processing for "natural products." Careful consumers should also ask how the digestion part of the process affects the product's bioactivity and how impurities are removed. Are heat or chemicals used? If digestion and/or sterilization adversely affects the active proteins, the substance will most likely have no efficacy. If, as is often the case, sterilization is achieved by irradiation, much, if not all, of the originally active antiangiogenic protein will be denatured.

Consumers should also be aware of some questionable advertising gimmicks. A co-owner of one large and well-known food supplement company actually said to me, "We advertise so heavily, we could sell horse manure and get away with it."

When an ad says the product is "further processed to produce a denser, granular consistency to assure maximum concentration for encapsulation," it means nothing more than changing the grind. In other words, the ad is using a lot of impressive words without much meaning. And what about the product that claims to be processed so that it is low in fat? Consumers would do well to ask where the fat came from in the first place. It is a well-known fact that no fat clings to the cartilage in sharks. Researchers began using shark cartilage instead of bovine cartilage because the lack of fat in the former eliminated the need for processing that could denature the active proteins (see *Bovine Cartilage versus Shark Cartilage* beginning on page 132).

Another ad for a brand of shark cartilage claims the product is a "synergistically blended herb formula for even greater bioavailability and assimilation resulting in a more complete product." I'd like to know what research has shown that the addition of herbs provides for greater bioavailability? Is it possible that someone in the advertising business believes that words such as "synergistically" and "herb formula" have magic properties that can sway consumers?

The term "mucopolysaccharides" is a real buzzword in the health field. Though widely used, this term is rarely understood. Many of the copycat products use the term "high" or "highest" in mucopolysaccharides. As a scientist, I have to scratch my head and question the intent. Mucopolysaccharides are credited with stimulating the immune system, and I believe they do. But, since their presence is very difficult to assay, we cannot assume that simply because a substance is high in carbohydrate—often dextrin—it is high in mucopolysaccharides.

The most dangerous "gimmick" from the point of view of

the patient seeking help, however, is the implication that "high in protein" means high in antiangiogenic activity. This is simply not true. The protein fibers in shark cartilage contain much, if not all, of the antiangiogenic activity. Protein derived from gelatin or from uncleaned shark meat or from horses' hooves has no antiangiogenic properties. If a product contained more fibers from shark fin, it would certainly be more effective, but at $200 to $300 for a few ounces of such fibers, I find it economically unfeasible—yet that's the implication on some labels. If the percentage of protein on the bottle can be misleading, a consumer's only insurance is the reputation of the product. Your best protection is to buy shark cartilage products that have shown positive results in clinical trials. Call the various manufacturers and ask if their products have been used in clinical trials. For further information, see "What to Look for When Buying Shark Cartilage" beginning on page 194.

Shark cartilage manufacturers would do well to spend less time on advertising and more on quality control and research. We mustn't make claims without substantiation. We must be able to prove effectiveness. Too many alternative products have been consigned to quackery because there was no evidence to substantiate the claims. Indeed, the American Cancer Society points to a lack of demonstrable evidence as a sign of a "suspect" treatment. People in alternative medicine are also sometimes considered "flower children." To ensure being taken seriously, they have to nail down their approaches with hard science and solid business acumen.

I feel strongly that when human lives are at stake, manufacturers must do more than just say their products are the same as what Lane tested or that they get results "as shown on *60 Minutes*." They owe it to the public to do some clinical work to justify their claims. Just saying a product is "equal to or better than" is not enough; desperate people seeking a last resort or some measure of hope may take the word as gospel.

One such situation has recently come to my attention. I cannot say if the claims are real or false. All I know is that the claims are, to date, unproven in either clinical or anecdotal results according to the management with whom I spoke recently. A Canadian manufacturer claims that 7 cc (approximately 7 grams) of its frozen liquid product has an antiangiogenic effect equal to about 100 grams of whole shark cartilage. Out of curiosity, I sent a sample of this product to a well-respected analytical laboratory for assay of the content. Much to my horror, the product was shown to contain 99.27 percent water. Since the antiangiogenic activity is in the protein fraction and the product is not purported to be homeopathic, I find it very hard to accept that 7 cc of a 99.27 percent water product can contain enough protein to be effective. This product is, however, widely sold and is being recommended by many well-intentioned doctors of alternative medicine, who seem to be basing their suggestion on a good sales pitch. I hope I am wrong for the sake of the patients, but as of this writing, I am very concerned.

I am also concerned about the wholesale use of words such as "new and improved." One particular shark cartilage product that is produced in Japan is often touted as "improved." No clinical trials have been run with the product and laboratory analyses reveal that it is 45 percent dextrin, or almost half sugar. It is also important to note that this cartilage product is processed using a technique I abandoned years ago. This process, which is indeed effective in reducing the product's mineral content, removes much of its active protein as well. Consumers must be aware that chemical and/or heat processing, as used by this Japanese company, alters protein.

Yet another product is called "100 percent shark-fin cartilage." The manufacturer or marketing expert may be playing on the fact that the Chinese have long proclaimed the benefits of shark fins and are voracious eaters of shark-fin soup, which they believe is an aphrodisiac and an elixir of youth. Whether or not these claims are true, natives of China have a lower rate of several types of cancer than do Westerners. Is the shark cartilage company in question guilty of misleading advertising, or is it really using only the fins of sharks to produce its product? Prudent buyers of shark cartilage should wonder how a company can obtain enough fins at low enough prices to profitably market a product. Concerned buyers must also question what becomes of the rest of the shark. It's an ecological necessity for us to utilize our resources cautiously rather than waste them.

The issue of utilization rather than waste always makes me think of Native Americans and their relationship with the buffalo. Plains Americans depended on the buffalo for much of their existence. Buffalo meat provided food, the hide was used for clothing and shoes, the bones were used to make sewing needles, and the animals' sinews became the thread. Fat from the animals was pounded together with berries and dried strips of meat to make pemmican (a trail food). The buffalo did not become an endangered species because of the natives that so relied upon it. The buffalo's existence was threatened by European settlers who wantonly destroyed the animals.

Scientific discoveries and media attention have prompted thousands of Americans to buy shark cartilage. I obviously understand and support the notion of capitalism, but it is totally unacceptable to use my work in an effort to take advantage of desperate people. It's hard to imagine anyone in a more vulnerable situation than a terminal cancer patient. I feel any individual or company who knowingly takes advantage of people in this situation is the lowest form of life.

The most horrific case of this kind of consumer fraud was reported in the British periodical *New Statesman and Society* in February 1994. Keith Banister, a British marine biologist and professor at the University of Kent, examined cartilage being distributed by one health-care professional. Dr. Banister said he could not find any shark cartilage in the product: "There was no sign anywhere of any cellular structure that would be detectable as cartilage."

And the problem goes beyond the hurting of those who are buying inferior products. Copycat products actually threaten the very existence of shark cartilage as a food supplement and a therapy.

INFERIOR PRODUCTS THREATEN THE GOOD

Copycat products that employ misleading advertising or are poorly processed pose a threat to the availability of shark cartilage products in general. The Food and Drug Administration (FDA) would invoke a Class I product recall if a product were contaminated and, therefore, posed a risk of serious health problems or even death. A Class II recall would result if a product posed the risk of a temporary health problem. Misleading advertising or products that are processed in ways that render the protein inactive might precipitate a Class III recall. In this case, the product is deemed to have violated FDA regulations regarding such things as truth in labeling.

Inferior copycat products might undermine my attempts to convince the "powers that be" of shark cartilage's efficacy. If a copycat product is processed so that the active protein or proteins are rendered inactive, the product will not be effective. Tragically, a poorly processed and, therefore, underpotent product might contribute to someone's death.

Such products also jeopardize the availability of shark cartilage products in general. When people talk about their experiences with shark cartilage products, they may not specify the name of the product that was found to be ineffective. You know how these conversations go: "Oh, shark cartilage? I tried it. That was nothing but media hype. It didn't help me at all." Even if the product name is mentioned, people may not remember it and may begin to believe that shark cartilage has no therapeutic effects. Some may even complain to the FDA. Consumers and the FDA may throw out the baby with the bath water. Before you know it, the products that do work will no longer be on the market. The publicity associated with a Class I or II recall will assuredly hurt even the "good" products. Furthermore, there is the risk that the FDA would recall all shark cartilage products if it were not clear which one had caused the problem.

One person who has voiced his concern is Sam Negaran, vitamin buyer for the Granary Health-Food Store in Sarasota, Florida. He is very concerned that people won't be able to get what they want. Those who feel they are getting successful results from shark cartilage will be forced to give up an alternative form of medicine in which they believe.

It appears that some unscrupulous businessmen are indeed producing products that are not properly processed and are even contaminated. Biological assays of these products reveal dangerously high levels of bacteria, a sign of spoilage. The previously mentioned frozen liquid cartilage produced in Canada is potentially dangerous since thawing and refreezing create an ideal medium for bacteria growth. If contaminants are shown to pose a health risk, the FDA will move quickly to pull the tainted products off the market.

BREAKTHROUGH IN PRODUCT DEVELOPMENT

Many believe that the discovery of shark cartilage as a therapeutic agent is a breakthrough in cancer treatment. Now that breakthrough has been joined by a revolutionary technological advance in processing.

For ages, shark cartilage has been eaten by the Chinese in the form of shark-fin soup. The Chinese "processed" the fins by drying them in the sun for about a week. Many companies marketing shark cartilage are using this same less-than-perfect technique. Imagine what happens to a moist protein product that lies in the sun for days; it's not surprising that cartilage processed this way is laden with bacteria.

Almost all quality shark cartilage products are produced from fresh or frozen cartilage that is cleaned of all meat and any bacteria. During this cleaning process, the protein-rich wings attached to the spine are often destroyed. And even if the cartilage is also sterilized (a process that might denature the active proteins), dead bacteria and the toxins they produce are still present.

Now, one company in Woodcliff Lake, New Jersey, is distributing a superior quality product that comes from Australia. The shark cartilage is processed using a revolutionary technique that eliminates the risk of contamination. Marine biologists, biochemists, and natural food scientists joined together and developed this new organic technology that eliminates the contamination without the use of chemicals or radiation. Shark cartilage is bathed in a naturally occurring liquid enzyme that digests or removes meat and contaminants from the cartilage without affecting the cartilage itself. The cartilage is cleaned in just two to three hours in stainless steel bins so that the product is truly untouched by human hands. Organic processing allows for the removal of unwanted tissue while preserving the soft cartilage wings, shown in Figure 11.1. Shark cartilage processed this way has more than 40 percent protein, which is up to 20 percent more protein than most shark cartilage products. This organically processed shark cartilage is one of the two products that have received FDA approval for clinical trials.

What to Look for When Buying Shark Cartilage

If you are interested in purchasing shark cartilage, you should know how to find the purest and most effective product. It is always a good idea to get a recommendation from someone you trust. You can, for instance, call (800) 510–2010 to ask about the products I am working with.

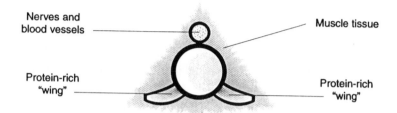

Nerves and blood vessels

Muscle tissue

Protein-rich "wing"

Protein-rich "wing"

Unprocessed Shark Cartilage

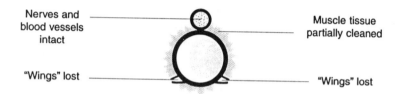

Nerves and blood vessels intact

Muscle tissue partially cleaned

"Wings" lost

"Wings" lost

Conventional Processing

Mechanical or hand cleaning scrapes away soft protein-rich "wings" but cannot remove all the meat from the cartilage. To remove the remaining meat, strong chemicals and bleaches are typically used, followed by aggressive sterilization methods.

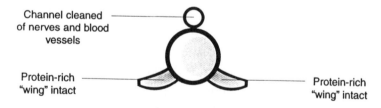

Channel cleaned of nerves and blood vessels

Protein-rich "wing" intact

Protein-rich "wing" intact

Organic Processing

A series of "organic" baths selectively removes unwanted tissue and saves the hard-to-clean soft cartilage "wings." This process is 100 percent free of chemicals, radiation, and ethylene oxide to ensure full product potency.

Figure 11.1. Shark Cartilage Processing Methods

When purchasing shark cartilage, you should keep the following points in mind:

❑ *Shark cartilage should be 100 percent pure.* Additives will only reduce the product's effectiveness. Manufacturers sometimes dilute their products to make them less expensive.

❑ *Shark cartilage should have no strong smell.* A mild fishy odor will, however, be apparent. A strong or foul odor may indicate that the raw material was spoiled or improperly processed. The product should not smell like ammonia or urine.

❑ *Shark cartilage should be off-white in color.* Tan, brown, or yellow cartilage may be the result of incomplete removal of meat. Residual meat increases the risk of spoilage and of high bacteria levels. If cartilage is pure white, it has probably been bleached, which may have rendered the product ineffective.

Remember, no one except the manufacturer is testing the product. The more discriminating you are, the safer you are.

WHAT COPYCAT PRODUCTS SAY ABOUT THE MARKETPLACE

Copycat products are a fact of life in the marketplace. I know an entrepreneur who doesn't even bother with patents anymore. His theory is "Get in. Advertise big. Make your money before the imitators—here and abroad—get a piece of your action." The existence of copycat products, as well as their being accepted as a fact of life, speaks volumes about the marketplace.

Are copycat products inherently wrong? I don't think so. The more important question is whether the copy is made to capitalize on existing success or to improve an existing product. If you can build the proverbial better mousetrap, more power to you. If you can build it at less cost and make a bigger profit, that's what capitalism is about. But if you increase your profit without offering added benefit or, worse yet, if you actually impinge upon the quality or effectiveness of the original product, then you're practicing free enterprise without scruples. You may make a quick buck, but you—and your business—will not survive the long haul.

John Wilcox, Ph.D., director of the Center for Professional Ethics at Manhattan College, in Riverdale, New York, believes copycat products to be an example of the "ethics of the fast buck. These are people who don't give a damn about the consumer. Normally, this doesn't happen with large corporations. They won't touch copycat products with a ten-foot pole. It's not in their best interests. It's not conducive to long-range profitability."

There are those who would like to see more and more regulation of business to force it into behaving ethically. Can there ever be enough regulations to prevent business people from ripping off the public? Stop a company from tearing the fins off sharks and chances are the company will find another less-than-savory way to make money. Legislate against phony gold mines, and someone will come up with phony oil wells.

"No amount of laws or code of ethics will take the place of recognizing that the purpose of business is service to society," says Dr. Wilcox. "Profitability is a necessary condition for success, but it is not the business' purpose. Too many businesses confuse the two so that need becomes purpose." Dr. Wilcox believes, however, that this is changing as more and more businesses begin to institute vice presidents in charge of business practices. There is even an Ethics Officers Association. "We need to address the culture, to arrive at a time where we believe in doing right because it is right not because laws or guidelines require it."

Perhaps copycat products indicate an underlying principle of modern life: we are motivated as much by laziness as by greed. The work ethic seems to have been replaced by the principle of doing the least amount of work for the greatest return. The perks are more important than the job description. And what's the favorite topic of conversation of many Americans? It's how they have avoided paying the full amount of income tax they owe or how they get cable TV without paying for it.

IN CONCLUSION

The fact that you're reading this book indicates that you want to know more about shark cartilage. That's a good start, but it's only a beginning. You must become a smart consumer. The more you know about shark cartilage, the less likely you are to be taken advantage of. Ask questions. Is the manufacturer reputable? Has the cartilage been overprocessed? Has it been adulterated with fillers, flavor enhancers, or questionable additives? Does it have a foul smell? What color is it? Is the price too good to be true? Getting the answers to questions such as these will help you to make the right decision.

Over two hundred years ago, President James Monroe said:

> Only enlightened public opinion based on accurate information and full and free disclosure of facts and issues can provide protection in the marketplace and still offer the consumer a free choice of products.

I think he was on to something.

Conclusion

*The science of one generation is usually the fallacy of
the next.*
—Sir Arthur Conan Doyle

Since my first book came out, I have been privileged to
travel around the world (several times), lecture to audiences both large and small, and meet some very interesting and caring people. Among them have been physicians, alternative health practitioners, media people, politicians, religious leaders, and cancer patients and their families. As I traveled, I learned a lot from what I saw and from the people I spoke to. This time has been both exciting and gratifying.

I've been confronted by literally thousands of heart-wrenching tales of cancer-related woes—tales of excruciating pain, crippling frustration, and fatality. Meeting cancer victims and coming to understand their plight has strengthened my resolve to see that the truth about shark cartilage becomes known. I am more determined than ever to see that the question of shark cartilage's efficacy as a cancer treatment be answered once and for all.

Yes, my journey, thus far, has been one filled with a number of eye-opening experiences. And as this is the book's conclusion, I wanted to share some final thoughts and observations with you.

ON RESEARCH

Just think—President Nixon declared war on cancer in 1971. The costs of that war have been astronomical, whether measured in human suffering or in dollars. Billions of dollars have been spent by the government on research to find the causes of and cure for cancer. That's our money—your tax dollars and mine—that the government has been pouring into research conducted by the National Cancer Institute (NCI) and by investigators who receive grants from that institute. In addition, our health-care and insurance costs are high in order to defray the costs of both development and use of new techniques, materials, and medicines. And even though corporate leaders as well as elected officials have invested billions of dollars in support of highly trained scientists, a cure for cancer still eludes us.

For as long as I can remember, I have always felt that medical research was constantly moving forward—making great strides. I believed that there were people in charge of making smart, logical decisions. At least, that's what I thought. Over the last five years, as I have tried to bring shark cartilage to the attention of researchers and the government, my opinion has changed.

In *The Politics of Cancer: A Study in Chaos,* an exceptional feature-length documentary, a United States senator is asked about the government's role in fighting cancer. He somberly explains how he had lost a good friend to prostate cancer and now truly understands how terrible the disease is. With great pride, he says that his friend's death motivated him to sponsor legislation increasing the budgetary allotment for prostate cancer research. I guess if his friend had died of lung cancer, more money would have been allocated to lung cancer research that year.

What the heck is going on? Where is the leadership? What is our direction? Do we really make financial decisions about cancer research based upon who just died and from what?

There are hundreds and hundreds of large and small territories marked out in the world of medical research, and no one wants to give up an inch of his or her property. Instead of visionary leadership, we must face the short-sighted dictates of supervising bureaucrats, directors, and heads of departments. Ask any real scientist who is familiar with the game, and he will say that many advances are made in spite of what goes on, not because of it. Luck is good to have, but it is not a replacement for leadership.

As someone who has had numerous government doors closed in his face, I can talk from experience. Unless you are well entrenched in the medical research community, your ideas have little chance of being recognized. Worse, in almost all cases, any work done outside the establishment is treated with disdain, if not outright hostility. Remember when the extraordinary results of the Cuban studies were made known and people began calling NCI for more information? They were told that I was a "charlatan." The callers wanted and were entitled to more information. And even though I had earned a master's degree from Cornell University and a doctorate from Rutgers University, had been a vice president of the W.R. Grace Corporation and an American envoy appointed by President Reagan, I was being called a fraud by a voice on the phone who had never spoken to me or asked to see my records. How many good people who have made a contribution wind up in the same situation? Where is the logic? Where is the vision? Where is the simple common courtesy?

ABOUT OUR HEALTH-CARE SYSTEM

Some say that our present health-care system is broken—that it wastes money and it excludes too many people. Well, I can't argue with that, but I don't think that explains why the system doesn't work. The problem is a lot more subtle. From early childhood, we are taught to go to the doctor when we are sick. We go. The doctor runs some tests, does some evaluations, prescribes some medicine, and we get better. That's the basic routine. Unfortunately, as we get older, we discover that some of the health problems we encounter do not get better in spite of fancier medical tests and more sophisticated medicines. But even if we do not get better, we do find answers and some measure of help. "You have arthritis," says the doctor. "Even if we cannot cure the condition, we can certainly make you feel more comfortable." Many times the answer provided is not a cure but a palliative, something that lessens the symptoms—usually a pharmaceutical product. Day in and day out, physicians repeat the ritual of providing some type of answer when patients are in need. And if they don't have the answer, they recommend a doctor who may. You see, doctors are supposed to have the answer—not necessarily the cure, but the answer. And it is on that premise that our health-care system runs. We, as patients, automatically go back time and time again to doctors who are trained to provide answers. "You have cancer, this is the treatment. . . . You have endometriosis, here's what we can do." Oh, treatments may help to alleviate symptoms for a while, but all too often patients come back because the symptoms have returned. Conditioned as we are, we continue to go to the doctor—who else do we have?

One reason our health-care system has weaknesses lies in the fact that our system does not have answers to all of our health problems, and that we, as patients, refuse to recognize this situation. We would do better to invest our resources in preventative medicine to avoid health problems. When conventional treatments fail, patients who have been ill always come back once the symptoms return. As the ranks of people who are ill grow, the size of our health-care system increases. Even if few get better, who cares? Someone else is paying. Now that insurance premiums have skyrocketed, now that the costs of medical procedures and prescriptions have become punishing, and now that our government faces the prospect of running out of money to finance this fiasco, we all should care.

We need to learn as much as we can about our health-care options, both alternative and conventional. By reading, by talking with others who have had experience with the various approaches, by speaking to health-care practitioners—both alternative and mainstream—we can make the informed decisions that will best serve our health-care needs. The fact is there are effective treatments for our illnesses that lie outside the "system"—treatments that work better, cost less, and have fewer, if any, side effects. However, when we ask someone in our system about using these "alternative" treatments for our own problems, we often get funny looks. We learn that few of these treatments are covered by insurance plans. We are actually made to feel that we are doing something wrong. There is nothing wrong with us. There is, however, something wrong with a system that refuses to see beyond its own research.

ABOUT PERSONAL FREEDOM AND RESPONSIBILITY

Our country was founded to preserve personal freedom. Over the years, landmark laws have been enacted to guarantee this freedom. Through too many wars, good men and women have sacrificed their lives for it. Yet today there exists in our country an attitude that greatly limits our personal freedom, at times without our even being aware of its loss.

Maybe the following scenes sound familiar: After months of feeling poorly, you are told, "There is nothing really wrong with you." You accept your condition as normal. . . . After discovering a lump, you are told that chemotherapy is your next step. When you ask if there are any other choices, you are told, "Not really." You set up your next appointment. . . . When you complain about the side effects caused by the pills you are taking, you receive a sympathetic look—and a prescription for another pill. You go directly to the pharmacy.

Too many of us are eager to give up our right to participate in the improvement of our health. And why should we participate when the system always provides someone who's willing to do the job? Subtly, medical protocol replaces personal freedom. Little by little, we have handed over the responsibility for our health and the health of our loved ones to a system that is designed to completely take charge of our health.

Instead, I took charge. While the mainstream scientists worked on isolating, purifying, and synthesizing the active components of shark cartilage, I ran with *whole* shark cartilage. The researchers who worked with me administered the pulverized shark cartilage and—lo and behold—we did see a positive effect, first on mice and eventually on people. I accomplished what I set out to do and I'm damn proud of it. You can—and should—live your life the same way.

I think it's important that we all take our lives into our own hands. This is particularly important for victims of what is labeled "incurable" or "terminal" disease. If the terminally ill just lie down and accept the verdict, nothing can possibly happen, nothing can change. Doing anything is better than doing nothing at all. What do you have to lose?

But what can you do? First, recognize that there are choices—lots of choices both in conventional and alternative approaches. By knowing what they are, by becoming an active player in your own health care, you regain precious personal freedom. Does this mean you have to give up going to physicians? Absolutely not. It means you should share responsibility with your doctor for your own well-being. And if your doctor is not willing to listen, find one who is.

In my previous book, I said that change—real change—occurs when people get together and demand change. I believe that, in part, the reason for the growing use of shark cartilage in this country is that people are telling other people about its benefits. It is also due to the growing number of open-minded physicians who sanction its use, and to those cancer patients—and their families—whose lives have been improved and extended through the use of shark cartilage. To each and every one of you, I say thank you for helping get the message out. But our struggle is not over by a long shot.

The problems I pointed out earlier still exist. Our health-care system is failing, too many of us refuse to take responsibility for our own health, mainstream medicine can't see beyond its own walls, and few are willing to make meaningful decisions to change what's wrong. It will not be Republicans; it will not be Democrats; it will not be independents. You and I will make the changes. How? By taking back some control over our own health. By learning as much as we can about the various alternative approaches to health.

Make your position about improving the state of our health-care system clear to your elected officials. Whether it's to your town hall or to the White House, call, write, and vote for something workable to be done. Do you realize the power of such actions? Elected officials know that for every phone call and letter received, there are thousands of Americans who feel the same way. Your voice counts. You can also join groups. Network with others who feel as you do. Send a message that we need responsible leadership to expand our options, not to block them. We can make it all happen if we want to.

SOME FINAL THOUGHTS

In closing, I would like to address those critics who have accused me of offering false hope despite evidence to the contrary. Shark cartilage's potential as a cancer therapy rests on a theory postulated more than twenty years ago by one of the most respected researchers in this country—Dr. Judah Folkman of

Harvard Medical School. Back in 1971, he said that inhibiting the development of blood vessels could be a potential cancer therapy. Today, that theory is being called an "extremely hot topic" and is being investigated by scientists at the nation's most prestigious institutions—the National Institutes of Health, Scripps Institute, Northwestern University, and Harvard University—and by such leaders in the pharmaceutical world as Bristol-Myers Squibb. In addition, concrete evidence in support of Dr. Folkman's hypothesis has been provided by Drs. Robert Langer and Anne Lee of the Massachussets Institute of Technology who demonstrated that an extract of shark cartilage inhibited the development of blood vessels in rabbit eyes. And evidence that shark cartilage can reduce tumor growth in people has come from clinical trials in Cuba and the United States.

I believe that the evidence presented in this book will put to rest the criticism of false hope, a criticism too often wielded by those who offer little or no hope in return. Shark cartilage does offer real hope to those suffering from largely incurable diseases, and hope is a beacon that should never be ignored.

Hope raises the human spirit. It helps us make it through the hour, day, and week. It is the starting place for both man-made and spiritual miracles. It lightens the darkness of despair. If I have provided hope for anyone who was without it, I am grateful.

I do not know where my journey will take me, but I have hope for myself, for those with cancer, and, yes, even for my critics.

To get on the mailing list for the shark cartilage newsletter, to obtain the latest information on clinical trials, or to receive a free pamphlet on the sixteen most commonly asked questions about shark cartilage call 800–742–7534.

Glossary

AIDS (acquired immune deficiency syndrome.) A condition affecting the immune system, which fights infection. AIDS is thought to be caused by the HTLV-3 virus, transmitted through an exchange of bodily fluids.

Analog. Functionally similar but structurally different.

Angiogenesis. The development of new blood vessels.

Antiangiogenesis. Against the formation of new blood vessels.

Antibody. A protein formed in the blood in reaction to certain substances that it then attacks and destroys.

Anticoagulant. A substance that retards or prevents the clotting of blood.

Antigen. A substance foreign to the body that stimulates the production of an antibody.

Apoptosis. Programmed cell death.

Arterioles. Small arteries.

Artery. One of the large blood vessels that carries oxygenated blood away from the heart.

Arthritis. An inflammation of the joints.

Articular cartilage. The cartilage in joints.

Assay. An analysis or examination.

Avascular. Without blood vessels.

Benign. Not malignant, harmless.

Biological (noun). A substance that alters the body's response.

Biopsy. The removal from the body and microscopic examination of a small piece of living tissue.

Bovine. Pertaining to an ox or cow.

CAM. Chicken chorioallantoic membrane.

CAM assay. A form of microscopic analysis in which sections of chicken embryos are injected with a test substance to determine if vascularization is being inhibited.

Capillaries. The smallest blood vessels; they link arterioles and venules.

Carcinogen. A cancer-producing substance.

Carcinoma. A malignant tumor originally composed of epithelial cells.

Cartilage. Gristlelike supporting connective tissue.

Cartilage-derived inhibitor (CDI). An antiangiogenic material found in cartilage.

CAT scan. *See* CT scan.

CDI. *See* Cartilage-derived inhibitor.

Chondrocytes. Cartilage cells.

Chorioallantoic membrane. A fetal membrane formed by the close association or fusion of two other embryonic membranes (the chorion and allantois).

Collagen. The main supportive protein of bone, cartilage, and connective tissue.

Control group. The group in a study that is left untreated and used as a standard against which the treated groups are judged.

Controlled trial. An organized, directed study or experiment in which control groups are used.

CT (CAT) scan. A procedure combining an x-ray with a computer to produce detailed pictures of the body in cross section.

Cytotoxic. Poisonous to cells.

Dalton. A measure $\frac{1}{12}$ the mass of a carbon-12 atom.

Denature. To change the characteristics of a protein by heating it or treating it with a chemical agent so that some of its original properties are diminished or eliminated.

Diabetic retinopathy. An eye disorder associated with diabetes in which the small blood vessels that transverse the retina dilate and rupture, leaving residues that usually impair vision.

Digestion. The process by which nutrients are made absorbable. During the process, the nutrients are broken down to simpler chemical compounds.

Double-blind study. A study in which neither the researchers nor the subjects know who is and who is not receiving the substance being tested.

Edema. Swelling of body tissues as the result of being filled with fluid.

Elasmobranchii. Fish having skeletons composed of cartilage. These fish include sharks, rays, and skates.

Endothelial cells. Cells lining the circulatory system; capillaries sprout from these cells.

Endothelium. The layer of cells lining the heart and the vessels of the circulatory system.

Enzyme. A chemical substance produced in the body that speeds up or causes a chemical reaction.

Epidemiologist. A person who studies the causes, development, and spread of diseases.

Epithelial cells. Cells found in the covering membrane of most organs of the body.

Fibrinogen. A precursor for fibrous protein that is involved in blood clotting.

Fibrosis. The formation of fibrous tissue in response to injury.

Gavage. Introduction of nutrative material into the stomach of a living organism by means of a tube.

Gestation. The period of time required for an embryo to fully develop within its mother.

Heparin. An acid mucopolysaccharide that prolongs the clotting time of whole blood; occurs in a variety of tissues, most abundantly in the liver.

Histology. The study of minute anatomy; the observation through a microscope of normal and diseased cells and tissues.

Hodgkin's disease. A malignant disease characterized by the progressive enlargement and inflammation of lymph tissues, particularly the spleen.

IND. *See* Investigational new drug.

Infarct. An area of dead or damaged tissue resulting from the failure of blood to reach that part. Infarcts are commonly found in the heart muscle following heart attacks.

Institutional review board (IRB). A panel of people who monitor research projects at an institution such as a hospital or university.

Interstitial space. Space between cells.

Investigational new drug (IND). A substance the Food and

Drug Administration approves for use in clinical trials but not for commercial marketing.

In vitro. In glass; refers to experiments performed in artificial environments (test tubes or petri dishes) rather than on living organisms.

In vivo. Refers to experiments performed on living organisms.

IRB. *See* Institutional review board.

Ischemic. Characterized by the loss of blood supply, usually due to some damage to the blood vessels.

Isolated organs. Organs maintained outside the body.

Kaposi's sarcoma (KS). A form of cancer in which irregular-shaped tumor cells cling to the linings of small blood vessels.

Killed-virus vaccine. Dead virus given orally or by injection to stimulate the development of immunity to infection by that virus.

KS. *See* Kaposi's sarcoma.

Lumpectomy. Removal of a cancerous lump and the immediately surrounding tissue from the breast.

Lymphoma. Any abnormal growth of lymphoid tissue.

Macromolecule. A molecule in a finely divided state that resists sedimentation, diffusion, and filtration.

Macular degeneration. A condition in which the central portion of the retina (the macula) is damaged so that central vision is impaired, perhaps severely.

Malignant. Refers to runaway cell growth that crowds out normal tissues.

Melanoma. A dark-colored tumor of the skin that is usually malignant.

Metastasize. To spread to a distant site or sites from a primary point within the body.

Mucopolysaccharide. Any of a group of carbohydrates containing an amino sugar and uronic acid (a sugar acid); found to have an anti-inflammatory effect.

National Institutes of Health (NIH). A federal agency that conducts and supports biomedical research in its own facilities and through grants to outside investigators.

Necrosis. A condition characterized by the death of body tissues or cells that are still in place and surrounded by living tissue.

Neoplasm. A new growth in body tissues; a tumor. A neoplasm may be malignant or benign.

Neovascular glaucoma. Glaucoma (increased pressure in the eyeball that causes defects in the field of vision) caused by the development of new blood vessels at the edge of the chamber containing the aqueous humor.

Neovascularization. The formation of new blood vessels; a synonym for "angiogenesis."

NIH. *See* National Institutes of Health.

OAM. *See* Office of Alternative Medicine.

Office of Alternative Medicine (OAM). A branch of the National Institutes of Health established in 1991 to investigate or aid investigation into those health-care practices considered alternative or unorthodox.

Osteoarthritis. A degenerative disease of the articular cartilage.

Peptide. A compound of two or more amino acids joined by a particular chemical bond.

Peritoneal. Relating to the peritoneum (the interior of the abdomen); more specifically, the strong membrane that lines the abdomen and helps hold the internal organs in place.

Petri dish. A shallow glass or plastic dish with a loosely fitting, overlapping cover used for bacterial plate cultures and plant and animal tissue cultures.

Placenta. The tissue that is attached to the uterine wall through which the fetus is nourished from its mother's blood; afterbirth.

Plasminogen. An enzyme that converts the fibrin in blood clots to soluble products.

Portal vein. The vein that passes blood into the liver from the digestive system.

Primary cancer. The site at which a cancer occurred originally.

Prophylactic. Acting to defend against or prevent disease.

Prostate specific antigen (PSA). A protein produced by prostate tissue; its appearance in the blood at certain levels indicates the presence of cancer.

Proteolytic enzymes. Enzymes that aid the breakdown of protein.

Protocol. The plan or procedure of a treatment program.

PSA. *See* Prostate specific antigen.

Psoriasis. A skin disorder characterized by reddish brown patches that become covered with silvery white or grayish scales of dead skin that eventually drop off.

Pulverize. To grind to a powder.

Retention enema. A procedure in which fluid is introduced into the rectum, held for as long as possible, and then expelled.

Retina. A membrane lining the inside of the eyeball and connected to the brain through the optic nerve.

Rheumatoid arthritis. An inflammatory disease primarily affecting the joints of the body.

Rheumatology. The study of diseases that cause pain in the joints, muscles, or fibrous tissue.

Sarcoma. A malignant tumor on connective tissue.

Secondary tumor. Not the original tumor in a body.

Squamous-cell carcinoma. A carcinoma composed principally of immature or undifferentiated cells on free surfaces or lining the vessels of the circulatory system.

Synergistic. A combined effect that exceeds the sum of its parts.

Thrombosis. A condition in which a blood clot develops within a blood vessel.

Topical. Referring to the surface area of the body.

Tumor. A neoplasm; new tissue made of cells that grow in an uncontrolled manner.

Vasculature. System of blood vessels; blood network.

Venule. A small vein.

Vertebrate. An animal with a backbone.

Water suspension. Separate particles dispersed in water.

Xenograft. A procedure in which tissue is transplanted from one animal to an animal of a different species.

Bibliography

AARP Healthy Questions: How to Talk to and Select Physicians, Pharmacists, Dentists and Vision Care Specialists. AARP Health Advocacy Services, 1992.

Ackerman, N.B., R. Jacobs, E.N. Kroop, and N.D. Bloom. "Evidence that Epinephrine Acutely Redistributes Blood Flow to Experimental Intrahepatic Tumors." *Surgery* 105:213+, 1989.

Ackerman, Norman, and Roger Jacobs. "The Blood Supply of Experimental Liver Metastases VIII. Increased Capillary Blood Flow Within Liver Tumors With Administration of Epinephrine." *Microcirculation, Endothelium, and Lymphatics* 2:457–475, 1985.

Adler, Tina. "The Return of Thalidomide: A Shunned Compound Makes a Scientific Comeback." *Science News* 146:424–425, 1994.

Alpers, David. "Digestion and Absorption of Carbohydrates and Proteins." In *Physiology of the Gastrointestinal Tract*, Vol. 2, 2nd edition, Leonard R. Johnson, ed. New York: Raven Press, 1987.

"Alternative Medicine Chief Calls It Quits." *Science* 265:307, 1994.

Altman, Lawrence K. "Scientists Report Finding a Way to Shrink Tumors." *The New York Times*, December 29, 1994, p. 1.

————. "Sharks Yield Possible Weapon Against Infection." *The New York Times*, February 15, 1993, p. 8.

Angier, Natalie. "Where the Unorthodox Gets a Hearing at NIH: Head of New Office Tries to Add Rigor to Alternative Medicine." *The New York Times*, March 16, 1993, p. C1.

Arnot, Bob. "Meet *Good Housekeeping's* New Family Doctor." *Good Housekeeping*, May 1994, p. 44+.

Azizkhan, Richard G., Jane Clifford Azizkhan, Michael Klagsbrun, R. Clement Darling III, Evan Rochman, and Judah Folkman. "An Avascular Subpopulation of Chondrosarcoma Exhibits Limited Growth In Vivo and Is Unable to Stimulate Capillary Endothelial Cells In Vitro." *Surgical Forum* 32:424–426, 1981.

Beardsley, Tim. "Sharks Do Get Cancer." *Scientific American* 269:24–25, 1993.

Begley, Sharon, with Debra Rosenberg. "Helping Docs Mind the Body." *Newsweek*, March 8, 1993, p. 61.

Bier, Jerry. "Shark Cartilage a Cancer Cure?" *The Fresno Bee*, November 28, 1993, p. A20+.

Billings, Paul C., William H. St. Clair, Patricia A. Maki, and Ann R. Kennedy. "Distribution of the Bowman Birk Protease Inhibitor in Mice Following Oral Administration." *Cancer Letters* 62:191–197, 1992.

Blackadar, C. Brian, M.D. "Correspondence: Skeptics of Oral Administration of Shark Cartilage." *Journal of the National Cancer Institute* 85:1961–1962, 1993.

Blackburn, Maria. "Author Takes a Thrashing But Stands by Book on Cancer." *Burlington (Vermont) Free Press*, October 3, 1993, p. 3B.

Bloch, Richard, and Annette Bloch. "Positive Mental Attitude

. . . or Just Wishful Thinking?" *Coping: Living With Cancer,* November/December 1993, p. 21.

Blumberg, Neil. "Tumor Angiogenesis Factor: Speculations on an Approach to Cancer Chemotherapy." *Yale Journal of Biology and Medicine* 47:71–81, 1974.

Blumenson, Leslie E., and Irwin D.J. Bross. "A Possible Mechanism for Enhancement of Increased Production of Tumor Angiogenic Factor." *Growth* 40:205–209, 1976.

Boles, Mark. "Supplements From the Sea: Healing Down Deep." *Health Foods Business,* August 1993, pp. 36–38.

Brem, Henry, and Judah Folkman. "Inhibition of Tumor Angiogenesis Mediated by Cartilage." *Journal of Experimental Medicine* 141:427–439, 1975.

Brohult, Astrid. "Alkoxyglycerol-esters in irradiation treatment." *Advances in Radiobiology.* Proceedings of the Fifth International Conference on Radiobiology, Stockholm, August 1956, p. 241.

———. "Alkoxyglycerols in irradiation treatment." *Nature* 193:1304, 1962.

Brooks, Peter C., Anthony M.P. Montgomery, Mauricio Rosenfeld, Ralph A. Reisfeld, Tianhua Hu, George Klier, and David A. Cheresh. "Integrin $\alpha_v\beta_3$ Antagonists Promote Tumor Regression by Inducing Apoptosis of Angiogenic Blood Vessels." *Cell* 79:1157–1164, 1994.

Brown, Robert A., Jacqueline B. Weiss, Ian W. Tomlinson, Paul Phillips, and Shant Kumar. "Angiogenic Factor From Synovial Fluid Resembling That From Tumours." *The Lancet,* March 29, 1980, pp. 682–685.

Bucco, Gloria. "Shark Cartilage: Cancer Cure?" *Delicious,* July/August 1993, pp. 30–31.

Burdick, Daniel, M.D. "Building a Lasting Relationship With

Your Doctor," *Coping: Living With Cancer*, November/December 1993, pp. 22–23.

Burling, Stacey. "Shark Cartilage: Can It Reverse Cancer?" *The Philadelphia Inquirer*, June 14, 1993, p. F1.

Campbell, Duncan. "A Case of Shark Practice." *New Statesman and Society*, February 4, 1994, pp. 14–15.

Caplan, Arnold I. "Cartilage." *Scientific American* 25:84–94, 1984.

Cassileth, Barrie R., Edward J. Lusk, DuPont Guerry, Alicia D. Blake, William P. Walsh, Lauren Kascius, and Delray J. Schultz. "Survival and Quality of Life Among Patients Receiving Unproven as Compared With Conventional Cancer Therapy." *The New England Journal of Medicine* 324:1180+, 1991.

Chaudhury, Triptesh, Michael P. Lerner, and Robert E. Nordquist. "Angiogenesis by Human Melanoma and Breast Cancer Cells." *Cancer Letters* 11:43–49, 1980.

Clark, Charles S. "Alternative Medicine." *CQ Researcher*, January 31, 1992, pp. 75+.

Cohen, Samuel, Masae Tatematsu, Yoshitaka Shinohara, Keisuke Nakanishi, and Nobuyuki Ito. "Neovascularization in Rats During Urinary Bladder Carcinogenesis Induced by N-[4-(5-Nitro-2-furyl)-2-thiazolyl]formamide." *Journal of the National Cancer Institute* 65:145–147, 1980.

"Conference: Angiogenesis." *The Lancet*, June 5, 1993, pp. 1467–1468.

Cooke, Robert. "A Hope in Sight." *Newsday*, October 26, 1995, p. A7.

Crim, Joe William, and Robert A. Huseby. "Initial Events in the Vascularization of Day-Old Mouse Testes Implanted Into the Inguinal Mammary Gland Fat Pad: A Light Microscopic and Autoradiographic Study." *Microvascular Research* 12:141–156, 1976.

Crum, Rosa, Sandor Szabo, and Judah Folkman. "A New Class of Steroids Inhibits Angiogenesis in the Presence of Heparin or a Heparin Fragment." *Science* 230:1375–1378, 1985.

Culliton, Barbara J. "'Celus' Costly Stumble on IL-2." *Science* 250:20–21, 1990.

D'Amore, Patricia A. "Antiangiogenesis as a Strategy for Antimetastasis." *Seminars in Thrombosis and Hemostasis* 14:73–77, 1988.

D'Amore, Patricia A., and Michael Klagsburn. "Angiogenesis: Factors and Mechanisms." In *The Pathobiology of Neoplasia*, Alphonse E. Sirica, ed. New York: Plenum Publishing Corporation, 1989.

D'Amore, Patricia A., Alicia Orlidge, and Ira M. Herman. "Growth Control in the Retinal Microvasculature." In *Progress in Retinal Research*, eds. N. Osborne and J. Chader. New York: Pergamon Press, 1988.

Deleuran, Bent W., Cong-Qui Chu, Max Field, Fionula M. Brennan, Tracey Mitchell, Marc Feldman, and Ravinder N. Maini. "Localization of Tumor Necrosis Factor Receptors in the Synovial Tissue and Cartilage-Pannus Junction in Patients With Rheumatoid Arthritis." *Arthritis and Rheumatism* 35:1170–1177, 1992.

DiMasi, Joseph A. "Comment: Risks, Regulation, and Rewards in New Drug Development in the United States." *Regulatory Toxicology and Pharmacology* 19:228–235, 1994.

Dollinger, Malin, Ernest H. Rosenbaum, and Greg Cable. *Everyone's Guide to Cancer Therapy: How Cancer is Diagnosed, Treated, and Managed Day to Day.* Toronto: Somerville House Books Limited, 1991.

Durie, Brian G.M., Barbara Soehnlen, and John F. Prudden. "Antitumor Activity of Bovine Cartilage Extract (Catrix-S) in the Human Tumor Stem Cell Assay." *Journal of Biological Response Modifiers* 4:590–595, 1985.

Edington, Stephen M. "Angiogenic and Angiostatic Drugs: Reshaping Biotech's Future." *Bio/Technology* 10:981–985, September 1992.

Eisenstein, Reuben, Klaus E. Kuettner, Carole Neapolitan, Lawrence W. Soble, and Nino Sorgente. "The Resistance of Certain Tissues to Invasion." *American Journal of Pathology* 81:337–346, 1975.

"Enforcing the Food, Drug, and Cosmetic Act." FDA Consumer Memo, DHEW Publication No.(FDA) 74–1018, 1974.

Ezzell, Carol. "Cartilage Grafts Grown in Lab Dishes." *Science News*, April 25, 1992, p. 270.

"FDA Recall Policies." FDA Consumer Memo, DHEW Publication No.(FDA) 79–1064, 1979.

Ferguson, J.W., and A.C. Smillie. "Vascularization of Premalignant Lesions in Carcinogen-Treated Hamster Cheek Pouch." *Journal of the National Cancer Institute* 63:1383–1391, 1979.

Fessenden, Ford. "Calling Scientists to Account: Hearing on Breast Cancer Tests." *Newsday*, April 10, 1994, p. A6+.

"Field Investigations Launched by OAM." *AM* 1:1, September 1993.

Fink, John M. *Third Opinion: An International Directory to Alternative Therapy Centers for the Treatment and Prevention of Cancer and Other Degenerative Diseases.* 2nd ed. Garden City Park, NY: Avery Publishing Group, 1992.

Flam, Faye. "Chemical Prospectors Scour the Seas for Promising Drugs." *Science* 266:1324–1325, 1994.

Flint, Anthony. "Researchers Say Aid from Japan Falling." *The Boston Globe*, January 3, 1994, p. 27+.

Folkman, Judah. "Antiangiogenesis." In *Biologic Therapy of Cancer*, eds. Vincent T. DeVita, Jr., Samuel Hellman, and Steven A. Rosenberg. Philadelphia: J.B. Lippincott Company, 1991.

————. "How Is Blood Vessel Growth Regulated in Normal and Neoplastic Tissue?—G.H.A. Clowes Memorial Lecture." *Cancer Research* 46:467–473, 1986.

————. "Tumor Angiogenesis: A Possible Control Point in Tumor Growth." *Annals of Internal Medicine* 82:96–100, 1975.

————. "Tumor Angiogenesis: Therapeutic Implications." *The New England Journal of Medicine* 285:1182–1186, 1971.

————. "The Vascularization of Tumors." *Scientific American* 234:59–73, 1976.

Folkman, Judah, and Michael Klagsbrun. "Angiogenic Factors." *Science* 235:442–447, 1987.

Folkman, Judah, Robert Langer, Robert J. Linhardt, Christian Haudenschild, and Stephanie Taylor. "Angiogenesis Inhibition and Tumor Regression Caused by Heparin or a Heparin Fragment in the Presence of Cortisone." *Science* 221:719–725, 1983.

Folkman, Judah, Paul B. Weisz, Madeleine M. Joullie, William W. Li, and William R. Ewing. "Control of Angiogenesis With Synthetic Heparin Substitutes." *Science* 243:1490–1493, 1989.

Frampton, Chris. "Alternative Medicine Gets Official Study: NIH Assesses Unconventional Cancer Treatments." *Wall Street Journal*, August 2, 1993, p. 1.

Gallo, Steve. "Bristol-Myers Invests 160 Million in Biotech." *The Medical Herald*, December 1995, p. 24.

Gardner, Michael. "Intestinal Assimilation of Intact Peptides and Proteins." *Biology Review* 59:289–331, 1984.

Gelb, Lenore. "Hope or Hoax: Unproven Cancer Treatments." *FDA Consumer* 26:10–15, 1992.

Gimbrone, Michael A., Jr., Ramzi S. Cotran, Stephen B. Leapman, and Judah Folkman. "Tumor Growth and Neovascularization: An Experimental Model Using the Rabbit Cornea." *Journal of the National Cancer Institute* 52:413–427, 1974.

Glausiusz, Josie. "The Secret Healing Power of Sharks." *Discover* 15:86, 1994.

Goldsmith, Harry S., Ann L. Griffith, and Nicholas Catsimpoolas. "Lipid Angiogenic Factor From Omentum." *Journal of the American Medical Association* 252:2034–2036, 1984.

Gorman, Christine. "Medicine: How to Starve a Tumor." *Time,* January 9, 1995, p. 60.

Grey, Alicia. "Shark Cartilage Therapy." *Sunday Star-Ledger,* July 4, 1993, Section 6, p. 5.

Griffin, Marie R., Wayne A. Ray, and William Schaffner. "Nonsteroidal Anti-Inflammatory Drug Use and Death From Peptic Ulcer in Elderly Persons." *Annals of Internal Medicine,* September 1988.

Huseby, Robert A., Clyde Currie, Vincent A. Lagerborg, and Solomon Garb. "Angiogenesis About and Within Grafts of Normal Testicular Tissue: A Comparison with Transplanted Neoplastic Tissue." *Microvascular Research* 10:396–413, 1975.

Jacobs, Maryce M., Phillippe Shubik, and Robert Feldman. "Influence of Selenium on Vascularization in the Hamster Cheek Pouch." *Cancer Letters* 9:353–357, 1980.

Jackson, Dowdy, Olga V. Volpert, Noël Bouck, Daniel I.H. Linzer. "Stimulation and Inhibition of Angiogenesis by Placental Proliferin and Proliferin-Related Protein." *Science* 266:1581, 1994.

Kaiser, J. "Protein Nips Mouse Tumors in the Bud." *Science News* 147:262, 1995.

King, Robert P. "Cancer Cure May Be Fish Story." *Sarasota Herald-Tribune,* November 14, 1993, p. 1+.

Knighton, David R., Thomas K. Hunt, Heinz Scheuenstuhl, Betty J. Halliday, Zena Werb, and Michael J. Banda. "Oxygen Tension Regulates the Expression of Angiogenesis Factor by Macrophages." *Science* 221:1283–1285, 1983.

Korn, Peter. "The Testing of a New Breast-Cancer Drug." *Self,* July 1994, p. 74+.

Kull, Frederick C., Jr., David A. Brent, Indu Parikh, and Pedro Cuatrecasas. "Chemical Identification of a Tumor-Derived Angiogenic Factor." *Science* 236:843–846, 1987.

Kyozo, Tsukamoto, and Yukio Sugino. "Tumor Angiogenesis Activity in Clonal Cells Transformed by Bovine Adenovirus Type 3." *Cancer Research* 39:1305–1309, 1979.

La Chapelle, Jack V. "Cancer: Taking Charge." *AARP Bulletin,* March 1994, p. 8+.

Lane, Earl. "Science Fraud Hard to Detect." *Newsday,* April 10, 1994, p. A6+.

Langer, R., H. Brem, K. Falterman, M. Klein, and J. Folkman. "Isolation of a Cartilage Factor That Inhibits Tumor Neovascularization." *Science* 193:70–72, 1976.

Langer, Robert, H. Conn, J. Vacanti, C. Handenschid, and Judah Folkman. "Control of Tumor Growth in Animals by Infusion of an Angiogenesis Inhibitor." *Proceedings of the National Academy of Sciences* 77:4331–4335, 1980.

Langreth, Robert. "The Frog Treatment." *Popular Science,* August 1993, p. 58+.

Lasko, Keith Alan. *The Great Billion Dollar Medical Swindle.* Indianapolis, IN: Bobbs-Merrill Co., Inc., 1980.

Lee, Anne, and Robert Langer. "Shark Cartilage Contains Inhibitors of Tumor Angiogenesis." *Science* 221:1185–1187, 1983.

Leutwyler, Kristin. "An Inside Job: IL-12 Attacks Tumors on

Two Fronts, But Can It Win the Battle?" *Scientific American* 273:24, 1995.

Maier, Thomas. "Knee-Deep in New Cartilage." *Newsday*, January 23, 1996, p. B21+.

Mann, Charles C. "Press Coverage: Leaving Out the Big Picture." *Science* 269:166, 1995.

Marion, Georgette. "When Patients Ask About Shark Cartilage: An Update on Expectation and Reality." *Oncology Times* 16:35, 1994.

Marshall, Eliot. "A New Phase in the War on Cancer." *Science* 267:1412–1415, 1995.

———. "Peer Review: Congress Finds Little Bias in System." *Science* 265:863, 1994.

Marwick, Charles. "Alternative Medicine Office Urged to Act Rapidly." *Journal of the American Medical Association* 270:1513, 1993.

Matouk, George. "Scientists Hail New Cancer Study." *Manhattan Spirit*, May 13, 1993, p. 14.

Matthews, James. "Sharks Still Intrigue Cancer Researchers." *Journal of the National Cancer Institute* 84:1000–1002, 1992.

"Metastasis: When Cancer Runs Rampant." *Coping*, November/December 1993, p. 44.

Mitric, Joan McQueeney. "Sharks May Take Bite Out of Cancer." *York Sunday News*, May 2, 1993, p. C2.

Moses, Marsha A., Judith Sudhalter, and Robert Langer. "Identification of an Inhibitor of Neovascularization From Cartilage." *Science* 248:1408–1410, 1990.

Nakamura, Shuji, Shinsaku Sakurada, S. Zaki Salahuddin, Yasuaki Osada, Noriko G. Tanaka, Noritsugu Sakamoto, Masayasu Sekiguchi, and Robert C. Gallo. "Inhibition of

Development of Kaposi's Sarcoma-Related Lesions by a Bacterial Cell Wall Complex." *Science* 255:1437–1440, 1992.

"Neovascularization and Its Role in the Osteoarthritic Process." *Annals of the Rheumatic Diseases* 47:881–885, 1988.

O'Brien, Maureen. "New Book From Small Publisher Expounds Natural Cancer Remedy." *Publisher's Weekly*, November 16, 1992, p. 13.

Oh, Suk Y., and Lalita S. Jadhav. "Effects of Dietary Alkyl-glycerols in Lactating Rats on Immune Responses in Pups." *Pediatric Research* 36:300–305, 1994.

Oikawa, H., H. Ashino-Fuse, M. Shimamura, U. Koide, and T. Iwagushi. "A Novel Angiogenic Inhibitor Derived From Japanese Shark Cartilage (I). Extraction and Estimation of Inhibitory Activities Toward Tumor and Embryonic Angiogenesis." *Cancer Letters* 51:181–186, 1990.

Oliver, Suzanne. "Book Burning." *Forbes*, June 21, 1993, pp. 65–66.

"Oral Collagen and Rheumatoid Arthritis." *Science* 261:1657, 1993.

O'Reilly, Michael S., Lars Holmgren, Yuen Shing, Catherine Chen, Rosalind A. Rosenthal, Marsha Moses, William S. Lane, Yihai Cao, E. Helene Sage, and Judah Folkman. "Angiostatin: A Novel Angiogenesis Inhibitor That Mediates the Suppression of Metastases by a Lewis Lung Carcinoma." *Cell* 79:315–328, 1994.

Park, Robert L., and Ursula Goodenough. "Buying Snake Oil With Tax Dollars." *The New York Times*, January 3, 1996, p. A15.

Parkins, Troy. "Researchers Test TIMP-2 as Potential Tumor Terminator." *Journal of the National Cancer Institute* 86:174–175, 1994.

Paulson, Tom. "Shark Cartilage Promoted as Treatment for Cancer." *Seattle-Post Intelligencer,* February 11, 1994, pp. B1–2.

Phillips, JoAnna. "Shark Therapy Cartilage Used in Alternative Cancer Treatment." *Reno Gazette-Journal,* October 17, 1993.

Podolsky, Doug. "New Drugs for Once Unyielding Diseases." *U.S. News & World Report,* May 10, 1993, pp. 66–68.

"Progress Is Reported in Slowing Tumor Growth." *The New York Times,* October 23, 1994, p. L34.

"Protein Discovery: Blood Vessel Inducer Isolated, Cloned." *Chemical and Engineering News,* September 30, 1985, pp. 6–7.

Prudden, John F. "The Treatment of Human Cancer With Agents Prepared From Bovine Cartilage." *Journal of Biological Response Modifiers* 4:551–584, 1985.

Prudden, John F., and Leslie L. Balassa. "The Biological Activity of Bovine Cartilage Preparations." *Seminars in Arthritis and Rheumatism* 3:287–321, 1974.

Raloff, Janet. "AAAS: Shark Gut Goop No Snake Oil." *Science News* 145:143, 1993.

Rejholee, V. "Long-Term Studies of Antiosteoarthritic Drugs: An Assessment." *Seminars in Arthritis and Rheumatism* 17:35–63, 1987.

Rock, Andrea. "Breast Cancer: Cause vs. Cure." *Working Woman,* October 1994, pp. 33–37.

Rosen, J., W.T. Sherman, J.F. Prudden, and G.J. Thorbecke. "Immunoregulatory Effects of Catrix." *Journal of Biological Response Modifiers* 7:498–512, 1988.

Rosenberg, Debra. "Joint Studies." *Technology Review,* October 1992, p. 10.

Rosenthal, Sharon. "Steroid Substitute Has Promising Future." *The Medical Herald,* June 1994, p. 33.

Roth, Sanford H. "Nonsteroidal Anti-Inflammatory Drugs: Gastropathy, Deaths, and Medical Practice." *Annals of Internal Medicine* 109:353–354, 1988.

Salmon, J. Warren, ed. *Alternative Medicines*. London: Tavistock Publications Ltd., 1984.

Sanderson, Ian R., and W. Allan Walker. "Uptake and Transport of Macromolecules by the Intestine: Possible Role in Clinical Disorders (an update)." *Gastroenterology* 104:622–639, 1993.

Seetharam, Bellur, and David H. Alpers. "Cellular Uptake of Cobalamen." *Nutrition Review* 43:122–124, 1985.

———. "Protein Digestion and Absorption After Intestinal Resection in Rats." *Nutrition Review* 43:122–124, 1985.

"Shark Bites Microbe." *Time*, March 1, 1993, p. 17.

"Shark Cartilage Brings Hope to Cancer Patients." *Dayton Daily News*, May 9, 1993.

"Shark Cartilage May Help Put Bite on Cancer." *Natural Foods Merchandiser*, March 1993, p. 10.

"Shark Cartilage Products." *Vitamin Retailer*, March 1994, pp. 27–29.

"Sharks Provide Cancer Therapy Clues." *The Choice*, Fall 1992, p. 24.

Spingarn, Natalie Davis. *Heartbeat: The Politics of Health Research*. New York: Robert B. Luce, Inc., 1976.

Squier, Tom. "Tom Squier Looks at Books." *The Spring Lake (North Carolina) News*, June 30, 1993, pp. 5–6.

Stone, Richard. "Imanshi-Kari Case: Baltimore Defends Paper at Center of Misconduct Case." *Science* 269:157, 1995.

"Taxol Approved to Treat Ovarian Cancer." *FDA Consumer* 27:2, 1993.

Taylor, E. "ACS Survey Finds 9% of Cancer Patients Use Questionable Treatments." *Journal of the National Cancer Institute* 84:1002+, 1992.

Taylor, Rosemary. "Alternative Medicine and the Medical Encounter in Britain and the U.S." In *Alternative Medicines*, ed. J. Warren Salmon. London: Tavistock Publications Ltd., 1984, pp. 191–228.

Toledo, Lucas. "Gene That Triggers Cancer Growth Found." *The Medical Herald*, October 1994, p. 34.

Trapper, David, Robert Langer, A. Robert Bellows, and Judah Folkman. "Angiogenesis Capacity as a Diagnostic Marker for Human Eye Tumors." *Surgery* 86:36–40, 1979.

———. "Angiogenesis Capacity as a Diagnostic Marker for Human Eye Tumors." *British Journal of Experimental Pathology* 59:282–287, 1978.

"Treating Arthritis With Tolerization." *Science* 261:1669, 1993.

"Treatment IND for Multiple Sclerosis Drug." *FDA Consumer* 27:2, 1993.

Trentham, David E., Roselyn A. Dynesius-Trentham, E. John Orav, Daniel Combitchi, Carlos Lorenzo, Kathryn Lea Sewell, David A. Hafler, and Howard L. Weiner. "Effects of Oral Administration of Type II Collagen on Rheumatoid Arthritis." *Science* 261:1727–1729, 1993.

Underwood, Anne. "A 'Bad' Drug May Turn Out to Do Good." *Newsweek*, September 19, 1994, pp. 58–59.

Weidner, Noel, Joseph P. Semple, William R. Welch, and Judah Folkman. "Tumor Angiogenesis and Metastasis—Correlation in Invasive Breast Carcinoma." *New England Journal of Medicine* 324:1–8, 1991.

"Where Do IRB's Come From?" *AM* 1:2, 1994.

"Winning the War Against Cancer." *Woman's World*, October 26, 1993, pp. 6–7.

Williams, David G. *Amazing New Anti-Cancer Secret That's About to Take the World by Storm.* Ingram, TX: Mountain Home Publishing, 1993.

Wood, John. "Health." *Modern Maturity*, February–March 1992, p. 82.

About the Authors

Dr. I. William Lane received both his B.A. and M.A. in the field of Nutrition Science from Cornell University. He received his Ph.D. in Agricultural Biochemistry and Nutrition from Rutgers University. As a researcher, he studied and worked under two Nobel prize winners, Dr. James B. Sumner (winner in 1946) and Dr. Selman A. Waksman (winner in 1952).

Entering industrial research, Dr. Lane first worked in poultry nutrition in association with Frank Perdue and Donald Tyson. From poultry-feeding formulation, he moved into fish-meal production. Shifting into management, Dr. Lane joined W.R. Grace & Company as vice president, heading its Marine Resources Division, with operating plants in Peru, Chile, Brazil, Canada, and the United States.

After a successful decade in management, Dr. Lane was appointed by then-President Ronald Reagan to serve as a resource advisor to the newly emerging nation of Guinea. Upon his return from this mission, he became an independent consultant specializing in marine resources. Among his clients have been the United States Department of State, the Shah of Iran, the governor of Morocco, and Taiyo, the largest fishing company in Japan. For the past fifteen years, Dr. Lane has pursued his interest in the benefits of shark cartilage as a healing agent.

Linda Comac received both her B.A. and M.A. in English from the City University of New York. She has taught English, journalism, and creative writing for more than two decades. A freelance writer whose articles have appeared in newspapers and journals, Ms. Comac co-authored *Sharks Don't Get Cancer*, published by Avery Publishing Group in 1992. The mother of two sons, Ms. Comac is married to a biochemist who has been conducting biomedical research at major hospitals in New York City for over twenty years.

Index

AANP. *See* American Association of Naturopathic Physicians.

ACAM. *See* American College for Advancement in Medicine.

ACS. *See* American Cancer Society.

Adamis, Dr. Anthony, 151

Adelman, Dr. Neal, 89, 143

Adlersberg, Dr. Jay, 87, 88

AGM-1470, 117

AIDS, 51, 58, 108, 115, 125, 141, 149

Aiello, Dr. Lloyd Paul, 151

Alkylglycerols, 12

Allen, Bruce, 84, 109–110

Alpers, Dr. David, 158, 160, 162

Alpizar, Dr. Carlos Luis, 131

Alternative Medicines, 79

Alternative practitioners, 175–77

Alternatives newsletter, xi

Alzheimer's disease, 15

American Association of Naturopathic Physicians (AANP), 177

American Cancer Society (ACS), xiii, 64, 179, 189

American College for Advancement in Medicine (ACAM), 177

American Scientist, 66

Amino acids, 158, 159, 162, 187

Andres, Dr. Harry X., 135

Angeliti, Dr. Donald, 143

Angiogenesis,
  arthritis and, 126, 129
  conditions based on, 150–151
  definition of, 11
  metastasis and, 13–14, 111, 118–119
  studies, 8–9, 25, 33, 77, 91, 107, 111–117, 120

tumor growth and, 42, 146,
    149
Angiogenesis inhibitors
    arthritis and, 130
    available, 58, 111–112, 189
    body's resistance to, 92,
        174
    development of synthetic,
        15, 72, 73, 93
    shark cartilage as, 10, 14–15,
        63, 94, 103, 121, 136, 186,
        187
    studies on, 111–117
    thalidomide as, 114–115
Angiostatin, 111
Antiangiogenesis. *See* Angio-
    genesis inhibitors.
Antigens, 126, 161, 162
Arnot, Dr. Bob, 83
Arthritis and Rheumatism, 136
Arthritis, 9, 125–129, 154
    bovine cartilage and, 130–131
    chicken cartilage and,
        137–139
    shark cartilage and, xv, 7,
        17, 22, 34, 114, 131, 134,
        135–136, 139, 150, 151,
        158, 164
Arthroscopic surgery, 128
Aspirin, 127
Atiba, Dr, Joshua, 86
Atkins, Dr. Robert, 157
Autoimmune psoriasis, 34.
    See also Psoriasis.
AZT (Zidovudine), 51, 54

Ballenger, William, 59
Banister, Dr. Keith, 191
Barret, Stephen, 83
BBI. *See* Bowman Birk
    protease inhibitor.
Beardsley, Tim, 23–25, 27
Belmont Report, the, 53
BeneFin shark cartilage, 148
Biotechnology, 34, 107
Blackadar, Dr. Brian, 68,
    159
Bloch, Richard, 175, 182
Bothum, Davella, 84, 85, 86
Bothum, Wallace, 84, 85, 86
Botulism, 160
Bovine cartilage, 7, 10, 130–
    131, 132–134
Bowman Birk protease inhibi-
    tor (BBI), 160, 161
Brain cancer, 110, 174
Bradley, Bill, 99
Braun, Jonathan, 38
Breast cancer, 16, 74, 95, 99,
    108, 112, 145, 146, 149
Breast Cancer Action Group,
    88
Bristol-Myers Squibb, 111
Brocks, Dr. Peter, 42, 113
Brody, Dr. Douglas, 180
Brohult, Dr. Astrid, 12
Burke, Dr. Gregory, 47, 108
Burlington Free Press, 88
Bynum, Yoriko, 153–155

CA-125 test, 84, 85

CAM assay. *See* Chicken
chorioallantoic membrane
assay.
Calcification of joint cartilage, 22, 127
Calcium, 163
Cancer
brain, 110, 174
breast, 16, 74, 95, 99, 108,
110, 112, 145, 146, 149
cervical, 110, 146
colon, 10, 112
gall bladder, 180
kidney, 142
liver, 99, 110, 142, 145, 149
lung, 153, 174
nervous system, 145, 149–
150
ovarian, 10, 41, 52, 84, 85,
86, 98, 110
pancreatic, 10, 142, 149
prostate, 41, 74, 99, 102,
106, 108, 109, 110, 112,
146, 149
renal, 149
sarcoma, 10, 54, 58. *See also*
Kaposi's sarcoma.
statistics about, 5–6
testicular, 10
types that respond to shark
cartilage, 146, 149–150
uterine, 6, 149
Cancer Control Society, 177
Cancer Letters, 26
Capillary endothelium, 7–8

Caplan, Dr. Arnold I., 24, 26,
27
Cartilage-derived inhibitor
(CDI), 15, 116, 119
Cassileth, Dr. Barrie R., 86
CDI. *See* Cartilage-derived
inhibitor.
Cell, 65
Center for Marine Conserva-
tion, 70
Cervical cancer, 110, 146
Chabner, Bruce, 67
Chemotherapy, 6, 10, 80, 81,
92, 108, 116, 118, 119, 135,
144, 153, 154, 156, 157,
164, 174
Cheresh, Dr. David, 42,
113
Chicken cartilage, 130, 137
Chicken chorioallantoic
membrane (CAM) assay,
14, 117, 121, 186, 187
Chinese National Cancer
Institute, 110
Chiou, Dr. George C.Y., 129
Chondrocytes, 128
Chondroitin sulphate A and
C, 136
Circulatory problems, shark
cartilage and, 156
Clinical trials, 31, 94–108, 157
Cuban, 6, 27, 28, 31, 39, 40,
57, 74, 80, 83, 86, 135, 146,
169–170, 206
FDA approval of, xvi, 3, 6,

27, 49, 53, 74–75, 108,
    110–111, 169
CNN, 17, 73
Code of Federal Regulations,
    53
Cognex. *See* Tacrine.
Collagen, 137, 158
Colon cancer, 10, 112
Colonic epithelium, 160
Comac, Linda, xv, 42
Crews, Philip, 5
Cytotoxic drugs, 92, 117, 164,
    181

Daiichi Pharmaceutical, 116
David L. Rike Cancer Center,
    87
Dayton Daily News, 42
Department of Health and
    Human Services, 65
Department of Health, Edu-
    cation and Welfare
    (HEW), 58, 59
Dextrin, 187, 190
Diabetic retinopathy, 34, 114,
    150, 164
Diagnostic tests, 171
Digestion, shark cartilage
    and, 158–163, 187
Dingell, John, 65, 67
Don, Dr. Philip, 99
Durie, Dr. Brian G.M., 10

Eighth International Breast
    Cancer Conference, 149

Eisen, Gail, 41
Ellis, Dr. Edward, 147, 148
Endothelial cell assay,
    186–187
Endothelial cell procedure,
    15
Endothelial cell stimulating
    angiogenesis factor
    (ESAF), 127
Endothelial cells, 92, 107,
    116, 121, 136
Enteritis, 150, 151
Epithelial cells, 162
Epstein, Dr. Samuel, 82
ESAF. *See* Endothelial cell
    stimulating angiogenesis
    factor.
Ether-oxygens, 12. *See also*
    Alkylglycerols.
*Everyone's Guide to Cancer
    Therapy* (Dollinger, et al),
    179
Eye diseases, 150–151
Eyewitness News, 21

FAIM. *See* Foundation for the
    Advancement of Inno-
    vative Medicine.
Fat, shark cartilage and, 188
FDA. *See* Food and Drug
    Administration.
Fernandez-Britto, Dr. José,
    xvii, 96, 98–99, 102, 103
Fibrinogen, 99, 102
Fisher, Dr. Bernard, 65, 66

Flam, Faye, 141
Fleming, Alexander, xi
Food and Drug Administra-
    tion (FDA), 34, 39, 45, 61,
    77, 80
  approval of clinical trials
    on shark cartilage by, xiii,
    xvi, 3, 6, 27, 44, 48, 58, 73,
    74, 78, 87, 108, 143, 149,
    152
  approval process of, 15,
    46, 49–54, 67
  marketing regulations of,
    16, 46–48, 192
  toxicity testing required
    by, 10, 60
Fordham, Sonja, 70
Folkman, Dr. Judah, xiii, 7, 8,
    14, 24, 34, 42, 62, 77, 91,
    92, 94, 112, 113, 115, 117,
    169, 205, 206
Forrest, Dr. John, 29
Forsythe, Dr. James, 82,
    180
Fox-5 Television, 2, 180
Foundation for the Advance-
    ment of Innovative
    Medicine (FAIM), 177
Fraud, scientific research
    and, 64–67
Fungi, 13

Gaby, Dr. Alan, 88
Gallo, Dr. Robert, 54, 58, 112,
    163

Gall bladder, cancer of the,
    180
Gannett News Service, 72
GAO. *See* General Account-
    ing Office.
Gardner, Dr. Michael, 159
General Accounting Office
    (GAO), 59
Gerson Institute, 89
GLACM. *See* Great Lakes
    Association of Clinical
    Medicine.
Glatstein, Dr. Eli, 73
Glenn, John, 59
Gonzalez, Dr. José, 87–88
Good Housekeeping, 83
Grane, Dr. Daniel, 128
Gravity's Rainbow (Pynchon),
    19
Great Lakes Association of
    Clinical Medicine
    (GLACM), 177
Green, Kyl, 56

Halfan, 52
Hamburg, Joan, 2
Harshbarger, John C., 24, 26
Health care, 201–203
Health Foods Business, 3, 184
Health insurance, 202–203
Health Insurance Associa-
    tion of America, 56
Healthcare Rights Amend-
    ment, 175
Heimlich, Jane, 178

Hemmings, Dr. W., 159
HEW. *See* Department of
    Health, Education and
    Welfare.
Hildenbrand, Gar, 89
HIV, 52, 115
Hivid, 52
Hodgkins disease, 33
Holistic Health Directory,
    177
Holland, Dr. James F., 21, 87
Holt, Dr. Stephen, 86, 99,
    122–123
Hypercalcemia, 163

IHC. *See* International Holis-
    tic Center.
IL-12. *See* Interleukin-12.
Imanishi-Kari, Dr. Thereza,
    65, 66
Immortalist, The, 43
Immunoglobulins, 162
IND status. *See* Investiga-
    tional new drug status.
Information services, 178
Ingber, Dr. Donald, 77
Insulin, 68
Interferons, 39–40
Interleukin-1 blockers, 129
Interleukin-12 (IL-12), 112
Interleukins, 39–40, 54, 57,
    112
International Association of
    Cancer Victors and
    Friends, 177

International Holistic Center
    (IHC), 177
Intestinal epithelium, 159,
    161, 162
Investigational new drug
    (IND) status, 3, 32, 48–49,
    50–54, 74, 78, 88, 108

Jacobs, Dr. Joseph, 55, 56,
    89
Jacobs, Dr. Roger, 64
Jain, Dr. Rakesh, 107
Jarvis, William, 26, 33, 88
Joint replacement surgery, 7,
    128
Jonas, Wayne B., 57, 89
Jones, Allen, 81
*Journal of the American Medi-
    cal Association,* 67, 89
*Journal of the National Cancer
    Institute,* 55, 68, 117

Kaposi's sarcoma (KS), 54,
    58, 59, 77, 108, 117, 149
Karnofsky Performance
    Scale, 96, 97
Kerbel, Robert S., 112
Kidneys, cancer of the,
    142
KS. *See* Kaposi's sarcoma.

LaChapelle, Jack, 168
Laetrile, 39
Lancet, The 33
Langer, Dr. Robert, xi, xiii, 9,

10, 15, 17, 26, 63, 92, 94, 120, 132, 169, 206
Langreth, Robert, 29
Lasko, Dr. Keith Alan, 61, 62
Lee, Dr. Anne, xiii, 9, 17, 26, 92, 132, 169, 206
Leprosy, thalidomide treatment and, 114
Leukemia, 33
Leukopenia, 12
Librax, 153
Liver, cancer of the, 99, 110, 142, 145, 149
Loratab, 153
Luer, Dr. Carl A., 25, 69–70, 72, 73, 120
Lung cancer, 153, 174
Lupus, 127
Lymph node swelling, 11

McCabe, Mary S., 25
Macromolecules, 162, 163
Macular degeneration, 114, 115, 141, 150, 151, 164
Madri, Dr. Joseph, 107
Magainin Pharmaceuticals, 13
Malaria, 52
Mankita, Jacob, 180
Market Place, 2
Mayo Clinic Family Health Disc, 150
Medical and Health Encyclopedia, 129
Medical World News, 81

Menendez, Dr. José, 96, 98–99, 146
Meshad, Dr. Michael W., 153, 154, 155
Metastasis, 13–14, 111, 118–119
Mexico, clinical trials in, 95, 134, 169
Milner, Martin, 110
Modulation, theory of, 102–108
Monsanto Chemical Company, 77
Mucopolysaccharides, 11, 72, 94, 132, 134, 135, 136, 187, 188
Multiple sclerosis, 158
Myelin, multiple sclerosis and, 137, 158

National Cancer Institute (NCI), 24, 25, 45, 46, 54–55, 57, 58, 61, 62, 65, 66, 67, 73, 114, 200, 201
National Center Against Health Fraud, 26, 33, 88
National Commission for the Protection of Human Subjects of Biomedical and Behavioral Research, 53
National Endowment for the Humanities (NEH), 59
National Institutes of Health (NIH), xii, xiii, 21, 41, 42,

45, 47, 53, 55, 56, 57, 58,
59, 60, 73, 75, 77, 85, 127,
163
National Science Foundation
(NSF), 59
National Surgical Adjuvant
Breast and Bowel Project,
65, 66
Natural Foods Merchandiser,
43
Nature, 77
Naturopathic Research
Laboratories, 32
Necrosis, 102, 103
Negaran, Sam, 193
NEH. *See* National Endow-
ment for the Humanities.
Neiper, Dr. Hans, 12
Neovascular glaucoma, 150,
151
Neovascularization, 8, 120
Nepron, 52
Nervous system, cancer of
the, 145, 149–150
*New Columbia Encyclopedia,
The*, 125
*New England Journal of Medi-
cine*, 8, 14
New Statesman and Society,
191
New York Times, The, 20, 21,
33, 34, 42, 112–113, 114
Newsday, 64, 65, 67
NIH. *See* National Institutes
of Health.

Nixon, Richard, 45, 58, 200
NOHA. *See* Nutrition for
Optimal Health Associ-
ation.
Non-steroidal anti-inflam-
matory drugs (NSAIDS),
127, 130
NSAIDS. *See* Non-steroidal
anti-inflammatory drugs.
NSF. *See* National Science
Foundation.
Nutrition for Optimal Health
Association (NOHA),
177

OAM. *See* Office of Alterna-
tive Medicine.
Office of Alternative Medi-
cine (OAM), 21, 55, 56, 57,
89, 90. *See also* National
Institutes of Health.
Office of Protection from
Research Risks, 53
Office of Technology Assess-
ment, 32, 34
Olarsch, Jerry, 32
Oncology Times, 86
Options (Walters), 37
Options and Health Care, 176
Oral tolerization, 137
Orcasita, Dr. José A., 131
Orloff, Dr. Serge, 131
Osteoarthritic synovia, 136
Osteoarthritis. *See* arthritis.
Osteoporosis, 53

Ovarian cancer, 10, 41, 52,
84, 85, 86, 98, 110

PAACT. *See* Patient Advo-
cates for Advanced
Cancer Treatment.
Pain, shark cartilage and, 96,
170
Pain killers, 7
Panama, clinical trials in, 95,
169
Pancreatic cancer, 10, 142, 149
Patient Advocates for
Advanced Cancer Treat-
ments (PAACT), 177
PDQ. *See* Physician Data
Query.
Peer review, 30–31, 35, 59,
63, 64–67
Penicillium notatum, xi
Pentosan polysulfate, 117
People Against Cancer, 57,
176
People's Medical Society, 176
Peptides, 158, 159
Peptone, 158
Physician, searching for a,
170–171, 175–179
Physician Data Query
(PDQ), 175
*Physiology of the Gastrointesti-
nal Tract* (Alpers), 158
Placental proliferin, 116
Planetree Health Resource
Center, 178

Plasminogen, 107
Platelet factor, 4, 116
PLF. *See* Placental proliferin.
Pluda, James, 115
Pneumocystis carnii, 52
Poisson, Dr. Roger, 66
*Politics of Cancer: A Study in
Chaos*, 200
Polypeptides, 93, 111, 158
Popular Science, 29
Portal circulation, 159
Portal vein, 160
PPNF. *See* Price Pottenger
Nutrition Foundation.
Pregnancy, shark cartilage
and, 156
Prescription Drug User Fee
Act of 1992, 52
Price Pottenger Nutrition
Foundation (PPNF), 178
Prostate cancer, 41, 74, 99,
102, 106, 108, 109, 110,
112, 146, 149
Protease, 158
Proteins, absorption of, 5, 56,
63, 67–68, 158–163, 189
Proteolysis, 162
Proteolytic enzymes, 93
Protozoa, 13
Prudden, Dr. John, xiii, 10,
17, 92, 129, 130
Psoriasis, 135, 145, 150, 164
Publishers Weekly, 43
Puccio, Dr. Carmelo, 133
Pynchon, Thomas, 19

Radiation, 6, 10, 12, 80, 108,
    119, 135, 156, 164
Ravis, Dr. Jacques, 131, 135
RDF. *See* Rheumatoid
    Disease Foundation.
Reagan, Ronald, 201
Real-Life Products, 144
Referrals, organizations that
    provide, 176–177
Rejholee, Dr. V., 139
Renal cancer, 149
Rennie, Dr. Drummond, 67
Reno Gazette-Journal, 180
Research grants, 75, 76–77
Retention enemas, 143–144
Rheumatoid Disease Founda-
    tion (RDF), 178

Salmon, Dr. J. Warren, 79
Sarcoma, 10, 54, 58. *See also*
    Kaposi's sarcoma.
Science, 5, 15, 22, 26, 30, 33,
    57, 58, 59, 77, 112, 116,
    122, 138, 141
Science News, 115
Scientific American, 23, 26, 27,
    28, 31, 88, 173
Scripps Research Institute,
    42, 43
Seattle Post-Intelligencer, 86
Selective perception, 19
Seligman, Dr. Barbara,
    144–145
*Seminars in Arthritis and
    Rheumatism*, 139

Senate Governmental Affairs
    Committee, 59
Shark cartilage
    absorption of protein in, 5,
        56, 63, 67–68, 158–163
    administration of, 142,
        143–144, 145, 146
    availability of, 170
    cost of, 156–157
    dosage for arthritis, 150
    dosage for cancer, 142–143,
        145, 149, 152, 154, 155, 156
    media reaction to, 37–38,
        86–87, 184
    physicians working with,
        178
    products available, 152, 155
    purification and processing
        of, 71, 72, 92–94, 186, 187,
        193–194, 195
    preventative use of, 151–152
    response rate of, 15, 174
    side effects of, 16, 143, 146
    synthetic forms of, 73, 93
    toxicity testing on, 74, 115,
        164, 169
    warnings against, 155–156
Shark cartilage products, 2,
    170, 184–193, 194, 196
Shark fin, 74, 189, 190, 193
Shark liver oil, 11, 12
Sharks
    cancer incidence of, 25
    endangerment of, 70–72
    health products from, 11–13

Sharks Don't Get Cancer (Lane & Comac), xv, xvi, 1, 18, 38, 41, 42, 43, 44, 47, 80, 154, 185
health market and, 2–3, 184
media response to, 1–2, 19, 38, 43–44
peer criticism of, 21–31
Shepherd, Steve, 38
Shur, Rudy, xv, 38
Simone, Dr. Charles, 25, 164, 180
60 Minutes, 2, 6, 24, 25, 30, 31, 38, 39, 40, 41, 42, 44, 58, 73, 86, 180, 184, 185, 189
Smith, Adam, 183
SP-P6. *See* Sulfated polysaccharide-peptidoglycan.
Spiny dogfish. *See Squalus acanthias.*
Standish, Dr. Leanna, 89
Stedman's Medical Dictionary, 91
Stern, Mark, 56, 57
Steroids, 127
Stetler-Stevenson, Dr. William, 62, 117, 119
Stracener, Dona, 153
Squalamine, 13
Squalus acanthius, 13
Sulfated polysaccharide-peptidoglycan (SP-P6, 117
Surgery, cancer, 6, 10, 80, 156, 164

Synovial fluid, 127

Tacrine, 15
Takeda, 77
Tamoxafen, 16, 98
Taxol, 16, 52, 54
Teff, Sister Michelle, 147, 148
Testicular cancer, 10
Thalidomide, 114–115
Thrombocytopenia, 12
Thrombospondin, 116
TIMP-2. *See* Tissue inhibitor metalloproteinase.
Tissue inhibitor metalloproteinase (TIMP-2), 117, 119
TNF. *See* Tumor necrosis factor.
Townsend Letter, The, 88
Trentham, Dr. David, 136, 137, 138
Triglycerides, 12
Tumor necrosis factor (TNF), 136
Tumors, 7, 8, 9, 14, 146–147, 163, 164

Uhle, Dr. Ivan P., 85, 86
Uterine cancer, 6, 149

Vascularization, 9, 22, 62, 146, 186
Vitamin A, 11
Vitamin Retailer, 184

WABC-TV, 87
Wall Street Journal, 55
Walker, Dr. Morton, 38
Wallace, Mike, 39, 40
Walters, Richard, 37
What Your Doctor Won't Tell You (Heimlich), 178
White blood cells, 12, 126
Wiewel, Frank, 57, 178
Wilcox, Dr. John, 197
Williams, Dr. David, xiv
Wolmark, Norman, 66
Woman's World, 164

Wong, Dr. Kin-Ping, 15
WOR Radio, 2, 157
Working Woman, 64, 82
World Congress of Anatomic and Clinical Pathology, 28

Yanes, Dr. Basel, 87
Yoshida, Dr. Kenshi, 110

Zasloff, Dr. Michael, 13
Zetter, Dr. Bruce, 157
Zidovudine. *See* AZT.

Other Avery Books of Interest

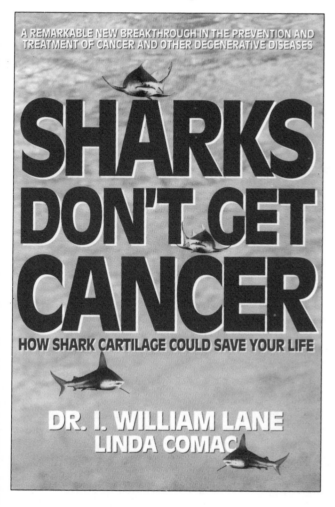

The Book That Started It All

SHARKS DON'T GET CANCER
How Shark Cartilage Could Save Your Life
I. William Lane and Linda Comac

In Sharks Don't Get Cancer, you will learn how sharks may be instrumental in overcoming a deadly disease—cancer.

In 1983, researchers at MIT released a study showing that shark cartilage can restrict the growth of tumors by stopping the development of the blood vessels that feed them. Researchers at Harvard Medical School found that by inhibiting angiogenesis—the development of a new blood network—one could prevent many devastating illnesses. Tying together the two important findings regarding cartilage and angiogenesis, Dr. I. William Lane recounts his own involvement in the search for a truly effective treatment of solid-cell cancers.

Shark cartilage may prove to be the first momentous step toward conquering cancer. Sharks Don't Get Cancer is the story of this amazing breakthrough.

Trade Paperback, $11.95

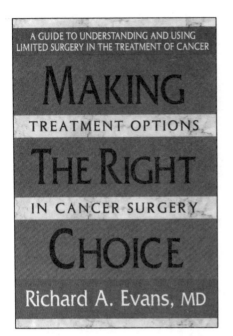

MAKING THE RIGHT CHOICE
Treatment Options in Cancer Surgery
Richard A. Evans

To answer the many questions that cancer patients have when faced with surgery, Dr. Richard Evans has written a complete and up-to-date guide to help them make the right choice—a choice based upon a clear understanding of the facts as they relate to today's research.

Dr. Richard Evans is a board-approved surgeon who views conservative surgery (removing the least amount of tissue possible) as a viable option for numerous types of cancer. He discusses how surgery is used as a treatment for cancer and why the profession has been slow to change its procedures. He then looks at cancer—what it is, how it spreads, and how it can be contained. In Section Two, Dr. Evans examines ten cancers that he thinks can be better treated with conservative surgery, from how each spreads to evaluations of treatments based upon the cancer's stages.

Trade Paperback, $14.95

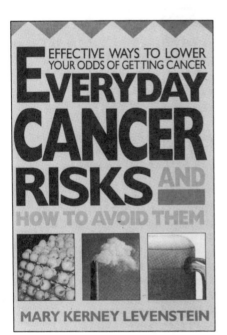

EVERYDAY CANCER RISKS
& HOW TO AVOID THEM
Effective Ways to Lower Your Odds of Getting Cancer
Mary Kerney Levenstein

Contrary to what you may have heard, not everything gives you cancer. But because of all the conflicting information, many of us feel confused and overwhelmed. The fact is that there are many things you can do to reduce your risks. Everyday Cancer Risks and How to Avoid Them is a practical survival guide for everyone who's willing to take back control of his health.

Thoroughly researched, this comprehensive book details all the major cancer-causing problems you may unknowingly come face to face with in your home, food, work place, and lifestyle. The author then provides a list of specific options from which you can choose so that you can avoid, remove, or greatly lessen the risk of exposure. Names of key organizations, associations, and product suppliers are provided, should more information be necessary.

Trade Paperback, $11.95

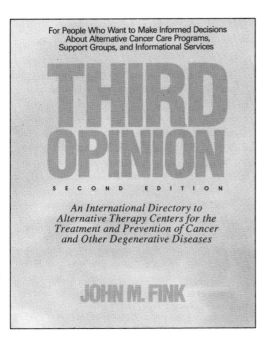

THIRD OPINION
An Int'l Directory to Alternative Therapy Centers for the Treatment and Prevention of Cancer and Other Degenerative Diseases
John M. Fink

Here, in an updated edition, is a comprehensive guide to the many alternative treatment centers located throughout the world. Everything you need to know—from addresses, phone numbers, names, and prices, to philosophical approaches and methods of treatment—is provided in a clear, easy-to-use format. Also included are the educational centers, information services, and support groups that may be of interest to the person looking for alternative or adjunctive therapy.

Trade Paperback, $14.95

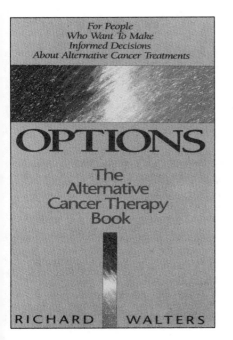

OPTIONS
The Alternative Cancer Therapy Book
Richard Walters

Alternative cancer therapies have helped thousands of "terminal" and "inoperable" cancer patients. Options covers a wide spectrum of available alternative methods of treatment from biologically based approaches to immune-enhancing treatments, dietary and nutritional regimens, herbal and plant-based remedies, bioelectric medicine, and adjunctive therapies, including information on recent experimental advances in cancer treatment.

This in-depth look at alternative therapies discusses how each approach works, explains the scientific rationale underlying each method, and presents clinical documentation of results. Options also includes guidelines for people considering alternative treatments and gives detailed information on referral services that help patients choose the combination of therapies best suited to their condition.

Trade Paperback, $13.95

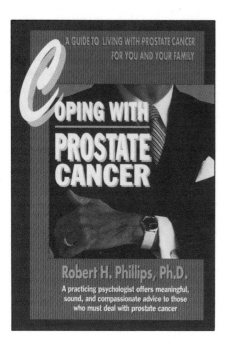

COPING WITH PROSTATE CANCER
A Guide to Living With Prostate Cancer for You and Your Family
Robert H. Phillips

It is estimated that by age eighty, almost all men will have some signs of prostate cancer. This new addition to the Coping with Chronic Illness series offers practical advice and comfort to the many men living with prostate cancer. The author answers all the important questions people have about this common disorder. He deals with the medical aspects of prostate cancer along with the many psychological and physical challenges involved. Included are sections on dealing with sexual relations, side effects of treatments, financial problems, relationships with others, and much more.

Coping With Prostate Cancer provides both the prostate-cancer patient and his family with the kind of practical advice they need at this most crucial time.

Trade Paperback, $11.95

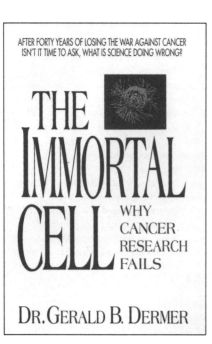

THE IMMORTAL CELL
Why Cancer Research Fails
Gerald B. Dermer

Dr., Gerald Dermer, cancer researcher, tells the amazing story of perhaps the biggest scandal in the history of science and medicine—of how billions of dollars in research money have been wasted because the research establishment has refused to improve its methods.

Most researchers have no experience working with human tumors. Instead, they depend on laboratory petri dish cells called cell lines for the information on human diseases. But cell lines are poor models for human cancer cells and can give incorrect information. In The Immortal Cell, the author explains why cancer research has failed to serve the public effectively.

Trade Paperback, $11.95